# FIRST AID



Editor: Karen Sullivan

Consultant Editors:
Dr Iain McNeil MBChB, MRCGP, DipIMC RCS (Ed)
Dr Michael Apple BA, MBChB, MRCGP

In accordance with
Resuscitation Council (UK) guidelines

BLITZ

The Publishers would like to thank the following for their help and enthusiasm during the production of this book:

Helen Allen, Edward Andrew, Melanie Aurora, Marina Borchardt, Kate Bouverie, Kate Brown, Holly Cayzer, Dr Mark Connaughton, Caleb Elliott and Edith Giffard, Angela Francis, Anna Gradara, John Grain, Sarah Griffiths-Rooney, Kourtney Harper, Barnaby Harsent, Rose Hudson, Doe Kan, James Kennaway, Katie Long, Tracy Lyons and Mel, Cecily and Max Mathias, Mark Mosby, Jane and Chris Parsons, Isabelle Rickard, Kathy Rooney, Peter Rowden, Diana Rutland, Kathryn Seabrook, Paul Sheehan, Tracey Smith, Pete Warren, Jane, Eleanor and Ferdinand Warrington, Sonja Welker, Andrew Whyte

Shoot Supervisors: Dr Iain McNeil, Doris Phillips
Photographers: Paul Lawrence, William de la Hey, Victoria Upton
Project Editor: Tracey Smith
Designers: Jessica Caws, Hugh Adams
Cover Design: Slatter-Anderson
Cover Images: Paul Lawrence, William de la Hey, Victoria Upton

Published by Blitz Editions
an imprint of Bookmart Limited
Registered Number 2372865
Trading at Bookmart Limited
Desford Road, Enderby
Leicester, LE9 5AD



A copy of the CIP record for this book is available on request from the British Library

ISBN 1 85605 383 0

10 9 8 7 6 5 4 3 2 1

Printed in Great Britain by Butler & Tanner Ltd, Frome

The publishers would like to thank the following
for their help and expertise:

British Allergy Foundation
British Association for Immediate Care
British Dental Association
British Diabetic Association
British Heart Foundation
British Red Cross
Help the Aged
London Fire Brigade
Medical Commission on Accident Prevention
Miscarriage Association
National Asthma Campaign
RAC Motoring Services
Royal Society for the Prevention of Accidents
St John's Ambulance
Surrey Ambulance Service
Sussex and Surrey Immediate Medical Care Scheme

# CONTENTS

# HOW TO USE THIS BOOK

This book is an indispensable guide to First Aid treatment for everything from travel sickness and bruises to life-saving rescue breathing and cardiopulmonary resuscitation (CPR). Each section is colour-coded for easy reference, and there is an extensive general index at the back of the book which will quickly guide you to the appropriate section. There is also a very useful symptoms index, so if you are not sure what treatment to offer, check here to see what the symptoms point to.

The first part of the book, **Emergency Situations**, is colour-coded **red**. Assessing the situation at the scene of an accident is explained and how to cope with multiple casualty incidents and traffic accidents. There are some tips on protection for the first-aider and health and safety signs to look out for.

The second part of this book, **Emergency Techniques**, is colour-coded **orange**, and covers all the essential techniques necessary for saving a life. Everything from the assessment of the casualty through resuscitation to treating bleeding and wounds is discussed here.

Part three is a step-by-step guide to treating **Emergency Conditions**, such as burns, choking and poisoning, all of which require urgent First Aid. This section is colour-coded **purple**.

In part four, which is colour-coded **blue**, you will find **Miscellaneous Conditions** such as bites and stings, travel sickness and nosebleeds, all of which respond to First Aid treatment.

Part five is colour-coded **turquoise** and contains general information on **Dressings, Bandages and Handling** a casualty.

Part six illustrates a **First Aid Kit**, which can be adapted to suit any needs. This section is colour-coded **green**.

The final section, **First Aid for...** is colour-coded **yellow**, and provides an excellent source of general reference information for treating babies and children, for drivers and passengers, people in the workplace, the elderly, sportsmen and travellers.

The symbol ☎ indicates when to call for an ambulance or other emergency services.

Each section is distinguished by a coloured tab.

Clear photographs illustrate the steps necessary for treatment.

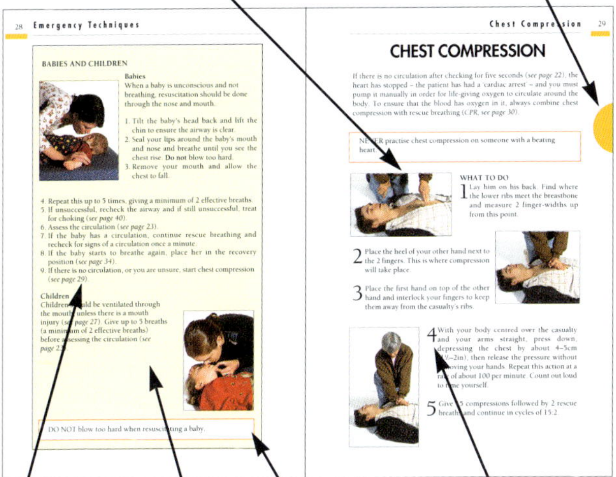
28 Emergency Techniques

BABIES AND CHILDREN

**Babies**

When a baby is unconscious and not breathing, resuscitation should be done through the nose and mouth.

1. Tilt the baby's head back and lift the chin to ensure the airway is clear.
2. Seal your lips around the baby's mouth and nose and breathe until you see the chest rise. **Do not** blow too hard.
3. Remove your mouth and allow the chest to fall.
4. Repeat this up to 5 times, giving a minimum of 2 effective breaths.
5. If unsuccessful, recheck the airway and if still unsuccessful, treat for choking (*see page 40*).
6. Assess the circulation (*see page 23*).
7. If the baby has a circulation, continue rescue breathing and recheck for signs of a circulation once a minute.
8. If the baby starts to breathe again, place her in the recovery position (*see page 34*).
9. If there is no circulation, or you are unsure, start chest compression (*see page 29*).

**Children**

Children should be ventilated through the mouth unless there is a mouth injury (*see page 27*). Give up to 5 breaths (a minimum of 2 effective breaths) before assessing the circulation (*see page 23*).

DO NOT blow too hard when resuscitating a baby.

Chest Compression 29

CHEST COMPRESSION

If there is no circulation after checking for five seconds (*see page 22*), the heart has stopped – the patient has had a 'cardiac arrest' – and you must pump it manually in order for life-giving oxygen to circulate around the body. To ensure that the blood has oxygen in it, always combine chest compression with rescue breathing (*CPR, see page 30*).

NEVER practise chest compression on someone with a beating heart.

WHAT TO DO

1 Lay him on his back. Find where the lower ribs meet the breastbone and measure 2 finger-widths up from this point.

2 Place the heel of your other hand next to the 2 fingers. This is where compression will take place.

3 Place the first hand on top of the other hand and interlock your fingers to keep them away from the casualty's ribs.

4 With your body centred over the casualty and your arms straight, press down, depressing the chest by about 4–5cm (1½–2in), then release the pressure without moving your hands. Repeat this action at a rate of about 100 per minute. Count out loud to time yourself.

5 Give 15 compressions followed by 2 rescue breaths and continue in cycles of 15:2.

Cross references direct you to other sections and pages in the book which will provide more information about the condition or treatment.

Essential guidance is clearly numbered in step-by-step form.

When babies and children require special care, the steps for treating them appear in a yellow-tinted box.

Vital warnings on what NOT to do in certain situations are shown in red boxes, and other options for treatment are given in green boxes.

# INTRODUCTION

First Aid is the first treatment or help given to a casualty either following an injury or at the onset of an illness, before qualified medical assistance is available. First Aid is one of the most important and useful skills we can learn, for all of us, at some point in our lives, are likely to be present at the site of an emergency. All it takes is a little confidence and knowledge to save lives, and that is what First Aid is all about.

First Aid is not complicated; there are a few basic rules that can be applied to most situations. The ability to preserve life, to prevent the casualty's condition from becoming worse and to encourage recovery is both rewarding and useful. Many lives are lost through ignorance and fear – you don't need to know much to make a difference; you don't need to be professionally qualified to save a life.

The aims of First Aid are simple:

- To keep the casualty alive.
- To prevent suffering.
- To prevent the injury or condition from becoming worse.
- To encourage recovery.

There are, however, a number of common mistakes made by people attempting to help. These are:

- Ignoring the absolute importance of the ABC of resuscitation *(see pages 10, 21)*, that is, checking the airway, breathing and circulation.
- A delay in getting help while treatment is given for trivial injuries or where an attempt to treat is unnecessarily prolonged.
- The use of tourniquets to control minor bleeding leads to the blood supply being cut off and limbs being lost.
- Attempting to treat serious injury instead of concentrating on the priorities. For example, if a person is bleeding extensively and not breathing, resuscitation takes priority over staunching the bleeding (*see pages 43, 58*). First Aid must be undertaken in a methodical way, following standard steps. The steps are easy to learn and essential for successful First Aid.

First Aid does not depend on fancy bandages or dressings. You don't even need to have a First Aid kit to treat seriously injured or ill casualties. What you do need is the ability to improvise, using the knowledge you have learned.

WHAT TO DO IN AN EMERGENCY

- Your first task is to assess the situation.
- Ensure there is no danger for yourself or the casualty.
- Get or call for help at the earliest possible opportunity, or see that someone else does it for you.
- Take charge – every emergency situation needs someone to assess and make decisions. Panic can ruin even the best-laid plans, and most people respond best knowing that someone is in charge.
- Deal calmly and confidently with any injuries; make sure that you have performed the ABC of resuscitation (*see page 21*).
- Reassure the casualty and everyone around you; do not leave him alone unless absolutely necessary.
- Arrange for treatment by a medical professional and make sure you are available to pass on any vital information.

The words and illustrations in this book will make it easy to learn the rules of First Aid. You will be able to practise these procedures no matter where you are, to recognise common injuries and conditions, to treat minor injuries and ailments at home, and to treat more serious conditions until help arrives. Emergencies will always happen; if you know the rules of First Aid, and how to apply them, you will be prepared to cope with the unexpected.

LEGAL CONSIDERATIONS

- No one has the right to touch (assault) or treat any one who does not wish it. Permission must be sought from the casualty.
- The unconscious casualty is deemed to have given their consent so that vital functions (i.e. the airway) are maintained.
- No one can be made to go to hospital – this may be refused together with examination and treatment.

# PRINCIPLES OF RESUSCITATION

The body requires oxygen for life. It is taken into the bloodstream through the act of breathing, and is vital for the energy processes necessary to living. When we inhale, oxygen and other gases are carried through the lungs to the bloodstream, which takes them to the tissues throughout the body; when we exhale, carbon dioxide, one of the body's waste products, is drawn from the bloodstream and expelled from the lungs.

The air that we exhale contains about 16 per cent oxygen, and that is why we are able to use that breath in rescue breathing, to save lives.

There are three main points to remember when assessing a casualty. They are called the **ABC of resuscitation.**

## *A AIRWAY*

The airway consists of the nose, mouth and windpipe. The airway must be clear in order to allow the essential passage of oxygen to the lungs. If it is blocked, a condition called hypoxia occurs, which means that the tissues in the body do not receive adequate oxygen and may die. The airway may be blocked by vomit, a small piece of food, the tongue falling back into the throat or a number of other things.

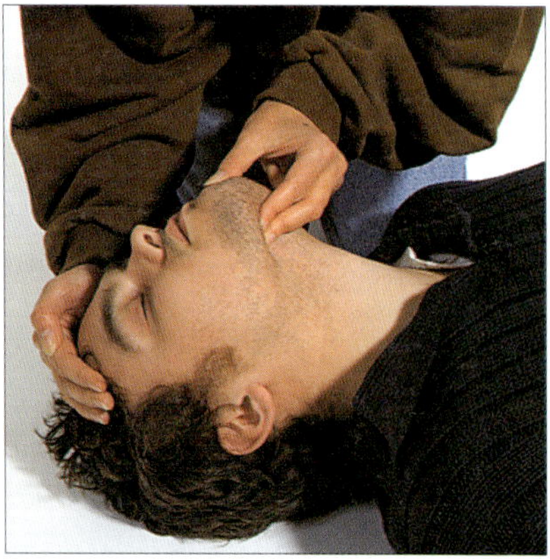

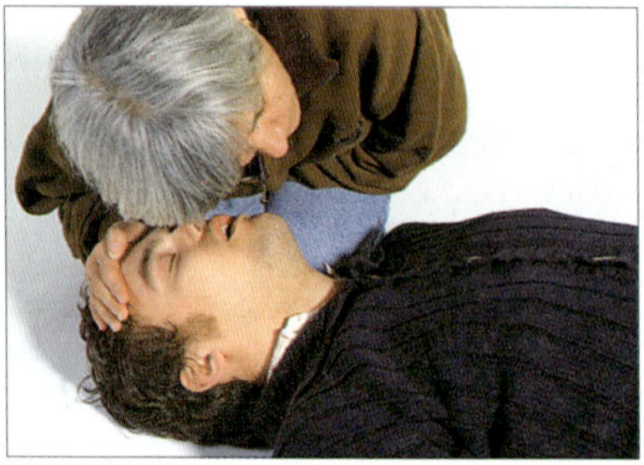

## *B BREATHING*

Breathing must take place in order for oxygen to reach the lungs. Breathing may not be possible if an airway is blocked. Many other things can stop a casualty from breathing – e.g. a head injury, drugs and cardiac arrest.

## C CIRCULATION

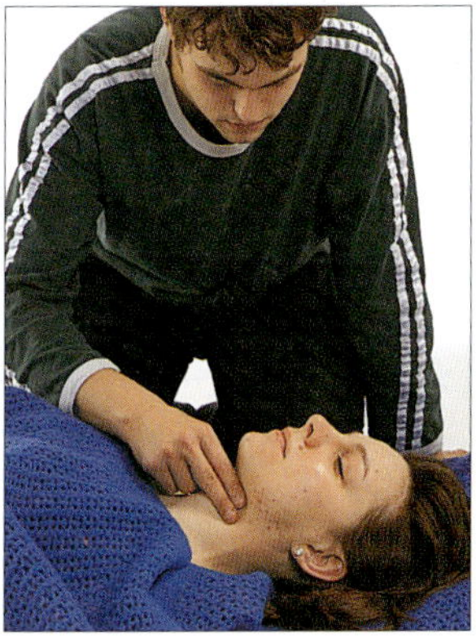

Blood must circulate around the body to carry oxygen to the tissues and carbon dioxide from them. If the heart is not beating, it may be necessary to apply pressure manually to pump the blood through the arteries (called **chest compression**, *see page 29*).

Without a constant supply of oxygen to the body, death will result. It is therefore essential that oxygen enters the lungs, and that the heart, which pumps the oxygenated blood throughout the body, is working. Cardiac arrest (the term used when the heart stops) means that the heart is unable to continue its action, so it must be done manually. Cardiopulmonary resuscitation, or CPR (*see page 30*), is rescue breathing and chest compression combined, which will 'buy time' by allowing the flow of oxygenated blood to be restored while waiting for professional help to arrive. It is very unlikely that CPR alone will restart the heart, which is why it is important to ensure the emergency services are called as soon as possible.

**In an emergency, the priorities are as follows:**

- **YOUR OWN AND THE CASUALTY'S SAFETY.**
- **IS THE CASUALTY CONSCIOUS?**

**FOLLOW THE ABC OF RESUSCITATION**

- **Is the Airway open?**
- **Is the casualty Breathing?**
- **Is there a Circulation? (In other words, is the heart beating? Is there a pulse?)**

**☎ CALL FOR AN AMBULANCE**

# EMERGENCY SITUATIONS

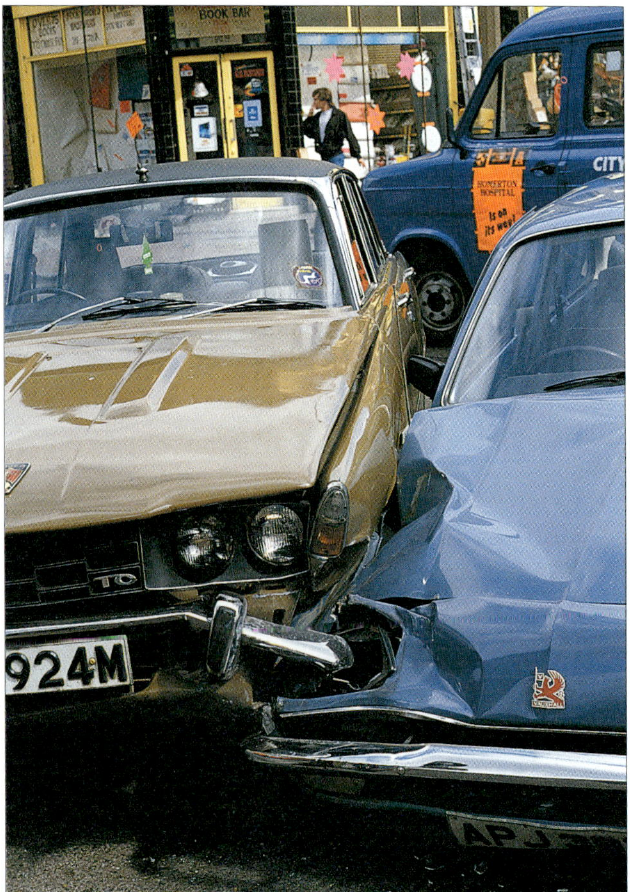

# ASSESSING THE SITUATION

Every emergency situation will be different. Helping someone who is choking in a restaurant presents a very different prospect from a multi-casualty traffic accident, but the skills required are basically the same, as is the order in which you should perform them.

There are some important things to remember in any emergency.

- Ensure there is no danger for yourself or the casualty.
- Find out what happened. How were the injuries received, and is anyone else hurt?
- Assess the situation and if the casualty is conscious ask her to describe her symptoms.
- Give emergency treatment to anyone who needs it. If there is more than one casualty, consider who to treat first (see below).
- ☎ Get help quickly (*see page 14* for tips).
- Employ the assistance of any other people at the scene to help clear the area, move the casualty, stop traffic or help to perform treatment.

## *Multiple Casualty Incidents*

Many accidents cause more than one casualty and it can be very difficult to assess who needs treatment first. Remember the following:

- ☎ Call for emergency help, providing as much information about the accident as possible. The emergency services will need this information to prepare for treatment, and to bring any specialist equipment that may be necessary.
- Casualties with less serious injuries should be moved from the immediate area and given quick advice about dealing with their own injuries (e.g. a bleeding hand can have a handkerchief wrapped around it which is then held by its owner). Even though they appear to be less seriously injured, try to get someone to be with them.
- Casualties who are unconscious should be assessed first. Follow the ABC of resuscitation (*see page 21*).
- Work calmly and confidently. You can't treat everyone at once and it is better to save some lives than lose them all.
- Assess conscious casualties next.
- Either make a mental list or ask someone to write down the order in which casualties have been treated, and the order in which you propose to treat the next ones, based on your assessment. This information will be invaluable to the emergency medical team before it begins work.

## ☎ Calling for Help

Emergency services can be called on **999** or **112**. These include the more obvious fire service, police and ambulance, as well as the coastguard, mine rescue, cave rescue, mountain rescue services.

> **Remember:** NEVER compromise your own safety in any emergency situation. However severe the casualty's injuries, it is vital that you ensure the area is safe before approaching.
>
> If there is an electrical problem or a gas leak, you may need to call the appropriate authorities. The emergency services operator should be able to do this for you or provide you with the right numbers.

- Provide the emergency services operator with as much information as you can about the situation – including your location, if known, the number of casualties, the cause of the injuries and any additional information, like a gas or chemical leak, or a risk of further danger.
- If there are any casualties, you must request an ambulance.
- Provide details about the injuries, including the sex, ages and the condition of any casualties.
- Always give your telephone number.

## Protection for the First Aider

- When giving first aid, be aware of the possibility of picking up or transmitting infectious diseases, such as hepatitis B or HIV.
- Cover your own cuts and grazes.
- Wear disposable gloves, whenever possible.
- For protection against infection you may use a disposable face shield for rescue breathing, if you have been trained to use one.
- If you can, always wash your hands before and after administering first aid.

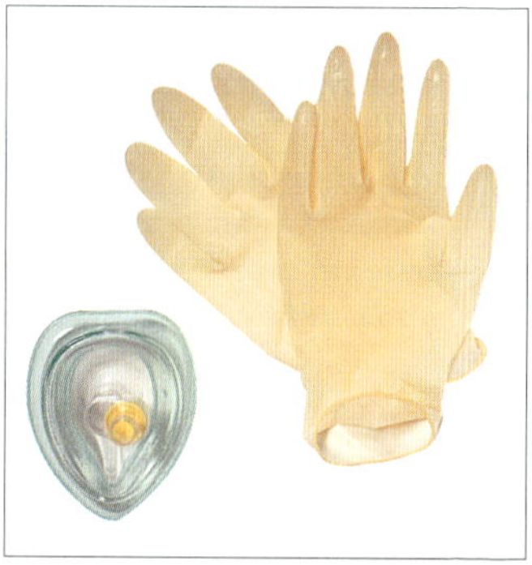

# Fires

- Do not attempt to put out a fire yourself, unless you have dealt with all casualties and the emergency services have been called. Then do so only if there is no risk to your own safety.
- If a casualty is on fire, wrap her tightly in a blanket or coat (anything which is heavy enough to put out the flames) and lay her down. Ensure that she is placed with the burns up (i.e. not lying on them).
- Cover your own mouth and nose with a handkerchief if there are smoke or fumes present.

**Fire Extinguishers**
*Back left*: Water (white): for use only on wood, paper, textiles and carbon-based materials.
*Back right*: Carbon Dioxide (black): for use only on petrol, oils, fats, paints and electrical hazards.
*Front left*: ABC Powder (blue): cannot be used on combustible metals.
*Front right*: AFFF Foam Spray (yellow): cannot be used on flammable gases.

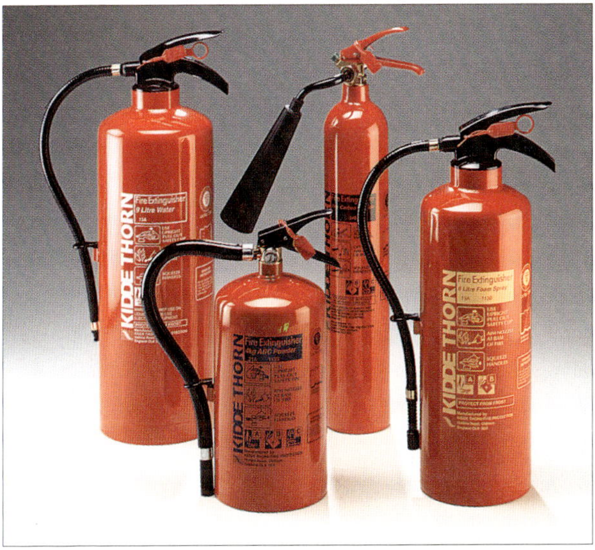

## *Health and Safety Signs*

Following are some of the health and safety signs to be aware of.

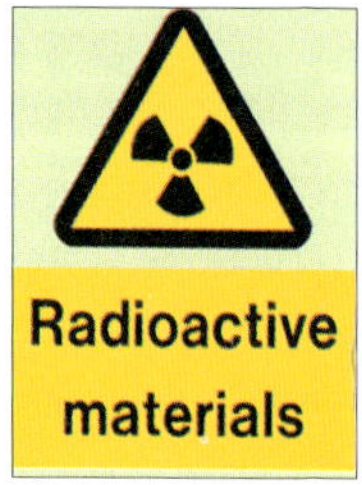

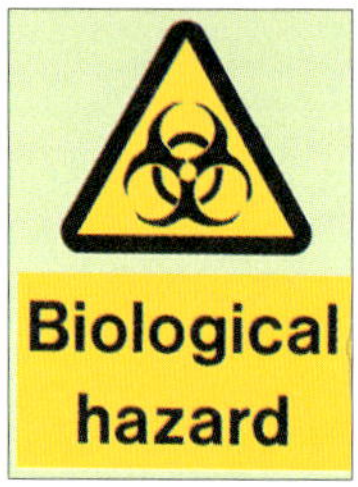


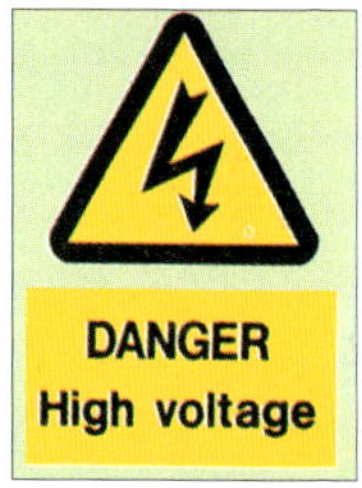


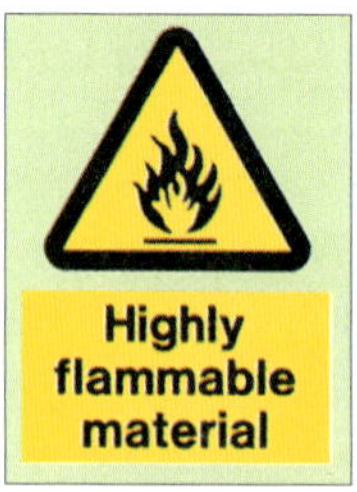


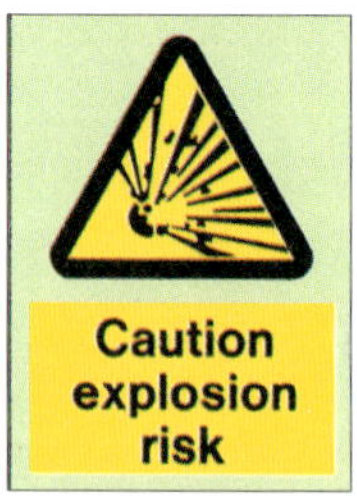

## *Traffic Accidents*

The most serious aspect of most road accidents is the risk of further injury or accidents from oncoming traffic. Your main priority will be to make the area safe for yourself, the casualty and anyone else sharing the road.

- Move your car clear of the accident unless it is one of the vehicles involved: turn on hazard warning lights.
- ☎ Call for the emergency services, indicating the number of casualties and the nature of the accident. If you have a mobile telephone, do not use it if petrol may be present.

- ☎ Attract the attention of any passers-by and ask them to warn other drivers. If you have not already done so, ask them to call for help.
- Set up warning triangles and lights in each direction. Allow about 50 metres (164 ft) or, on a motorway, 150 metres (492 ft) on either side to give other drivers a chance to stop.
- Turn off the engine of any car that has been involved, and if there are signs of fumes, flames or leaking petrol, stay clear until help arrives.

NEVER run across a motorway to get help or to provide assistance.

DO NOT move the casualty unless essential (e.g., there is further danger or a risk to the safety of someone else).

NEVER remove the crash helmet of an unconcious motorcyclist unless the airway is blocked.

WHAT TO DO

1. Ensure the safety of yourself and the casualty.
2. Check responsiveness by shaking the casualty gently and shouting.
3. Follow the ABC of resuscitation (*see page 21*) and be prepared to resuscitate (*see page 26*). Always assume there is neck damage. Support the neck.
4. Call for the emergency services and wait with the casualty until help arrives.
5. Walking injured and people who are not injured should be moved away from the scene.

If the casualty is trapped, do not try to free her. Wait until help arrives, but stay with her until it does.

When there are poisonous or corrosive substances involved in an accident, from a tanker, for instance, stay away from the scene and warn others to do so. Call for emergency help and give as much information as you can about the substance. Most tankers and lorries have details about their cargo on the side of the vehicle. ☎ There may be a telephone number to ring for further information. Pass this information on to the emergency services.

# WHAT TO DO IN AN EMERGENCY

**ADULTS**

↓

Approach SAFELY

↓

Assess CONSCIOUSNESS

↓

Shout for HELP

↓

OPEN AIRWAY
(*see page 24 if blocked*)

↓

Check BREATHING
for up to 10 seconds

Is casualty BREATHING?

**NO**

↓

Call for an AMBULANCE

↓

Give 2 effective RESCUE BREATHS (*see page 26*)

↓

Check CIRCULATION
for no more than 10 seconds
(*see page 22*)

**No circulation**

↓

Give 15 CHEST COMPRESSIONS
(*see page 29*)

↓

Continue in cycles of 2 rescue breaths : 15 chest compressions (or 1:5 if there are two first-aiders

**Circulation present**

↓

Continue
RESCUE BREATHING
(*see page 26*)

↓

Continue rescue breathing, rechecking circulation once a minute

**YES**

↓

RECOVERY POSITION
(*see page 34*)

↓

GET HELP

↓

**On return**
Monitor continued breathing (*see page 21*) and be prepared to do CPR (*see page 30*). Treat any injuries that require urgent intervention, e.g. bleeding/ fracture

## CHILDREN

↓

Approach SAFELY

↓

Assess CONSCIOUSNESS

↓

Shout for HELP

↓

OPEN AIRWAY
(*see page 24 if blocked*)

↓

Check BREATHING
for up to 10 seconds

Is casualty BREATHING?

**NO**

↓

Give up to 5
RESCUE BREATHS
(*see page 26*)

↓

Check CIRCULATION
for no more than 10 seconds
(*see page 23*)

**No circulation**

↓

Give 5 CHEST
COMPRESSIONS
(*see page 31*)

↓

Call for an
AMBULANCE

Take/carry casualty with you if you can, and continue CPR in cycles of 1 rescue breath to 5 chest compressions while waiting

**Circulation present**

↓

Continue
RESCUE
BREATHING
(*see page 28*)

↓

Call for an
AMBULANCE

Take/carry casualty with you if you can. Continue rescue breathing, rechecking circulation once a minute

**YES**

↓

Recovery position
(*see page 34*)

↓

GET HELP

↓

On return:
Monitor continued breathing (*see page 21*) and be prepared to do CPR (*see page 31*)

# EMERGENCY TECHNIQUES

In an emergency, the priorities are as follows:

- YOUR OWN AND THE CASUALTY'S SAFETY.
- IS THE CASUALTY CONSCIOUS?

**FOLLOW THE ABC OF RESUSCITATION**

- Is the Airway open?
- Is the casualty Breathing?
- Is there a Circulation? (In other words, is the heart beating? Is there a pulse?)

☎ CALL FOR AN AMBULANCE

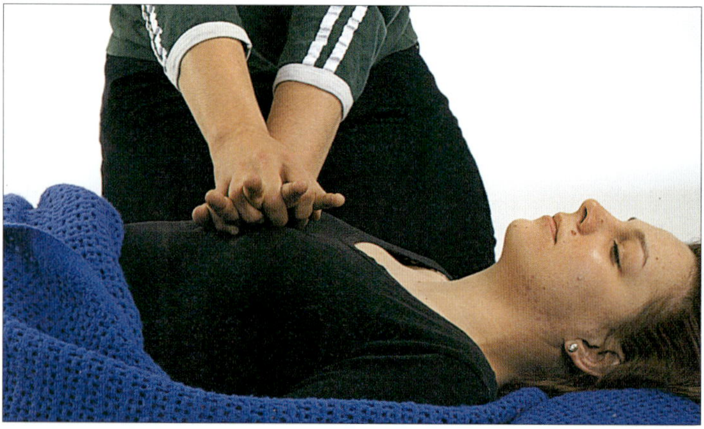

# ABC OF RESUSCITATION

The first step in any emergency situation is to ensure you are safe. The second is to assess the casualty's consciousness by shaking the shoulders and shouting at them. If they are unconscious, shout for help. The flow chart on pages 18–19 tells you what to do next, based on the outcome of each of your simple checks.

**REMEMBER THE ABC OF RESUSCITATION: AIRWAY, BREATHING AND CIRCULATION.**

## *1. Check the airway*

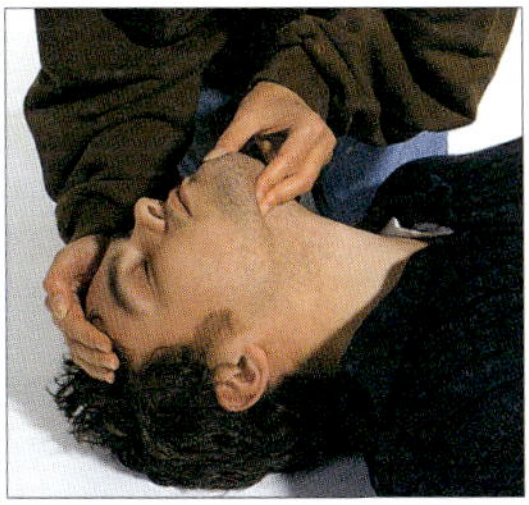

Tilt back the casualty's head and lift the chin in order to open the airway.

- Place one hand on the forehead and gently tilt the head back.
- Use 2 fingers of your other hand to lift the chin upwards.

This action prevents the tongue from falling back to block the windpipe.

BABIES AND CHILDREN
Tilt the head back and lift the chin. Do not tilt too far back as this may also cause obstruction to the airway in small babies.

DO NOT turn or tilt back the head if you suspect an injury to the neck. Simply lift the chin up and keep the head in position.

## 2. *Check for breathing*

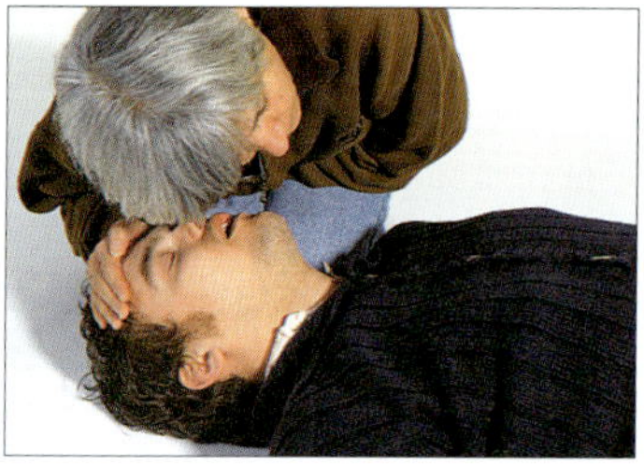

Is the casualty obviously breathing?

- Keep the airway open.
- Place your head above the casualty's face and look down the chest.
- Is the chest rising and falling?
- Can you feel any air? Can you hear any sounds of breathing?
- Look, listen and feel for breathing for up to 10 seconds.

If the casualty is not breathing, and you have someone else with you, send them to call an ambulance immediately, while you give 2 rescue breaths (*see page* 26). If you are alone and think the cause of unconsciousness is a serious injury, the casualty has been drowned or is a child, perform resuscitation for about a minute before leaving the casualty and ringing for an ambulance. Otherwise, if you are alone, leave the casualty and call an ambulance. Then return and give 2 rescue breaths.

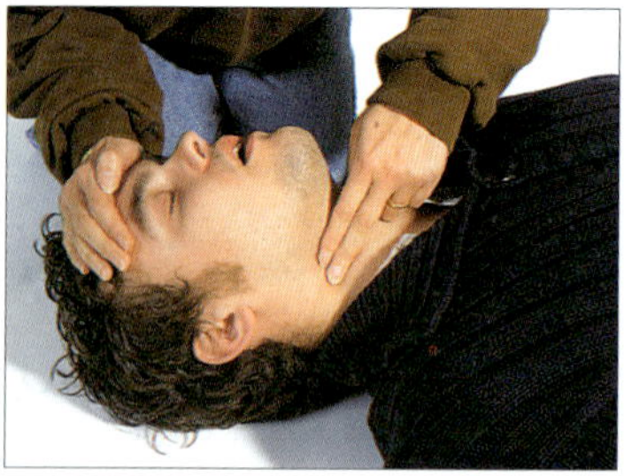

## 3. *Check for signs of a circulation*

- Look for any movement, including swallowing or breathing (more than an occasional gasp).
- Check for a carotid pulse for no more than 10 seconds using 2 fingers. You will find this in the hollow between the Adam's apple and the neck muscle.
- If there are no signs of a circulation, or you are at all unsure, begin chest compression (*see page* 29).

NEVER use your thumb to take a pulse since it has a pulse of its own.

BABIES AND CHILDREN

**To check for a circulation in a baby:**

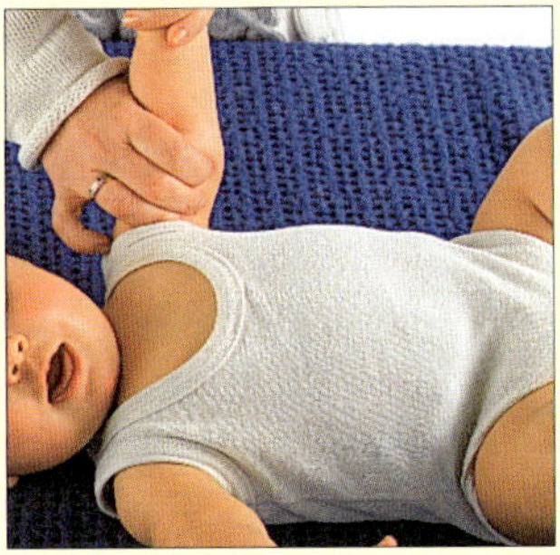

- Place two fingers on the inner aspect of the upper arm to feel the brachial pulse.
- Take no more than 10 seconds.
- Look for any movement, including swallowing or breathing (more than an occasional gasp).
- If there are no signs of a circulation start chest compression and combine with rescue breathing (CPR, *see page 31*).

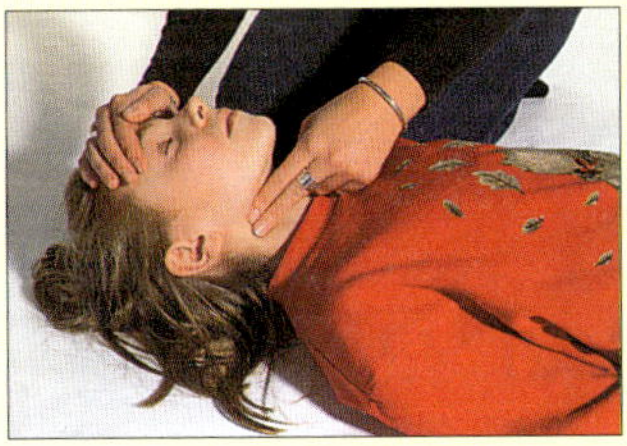

**To check for a circulation in a child:**

- Check the carotid pulse, as with an adult (*see page* 22).

# CLEARING THE AIRWAY

When the head is tilted back and the chin is lifted for the airway to open, breathing should be possible; therefore, the first thing to do with an unconscious casualty is to tilt the head back and lift the chin forward, if possible keeping him in the position in which he was found.

If the casualty is still not breathing, the airway may be blocked by vomit, broken teeth or a foreign object. If you are still unable to clear the airway:

WHAT TO DO

1 Turn the casualty onto his back, if he is not already in this position.

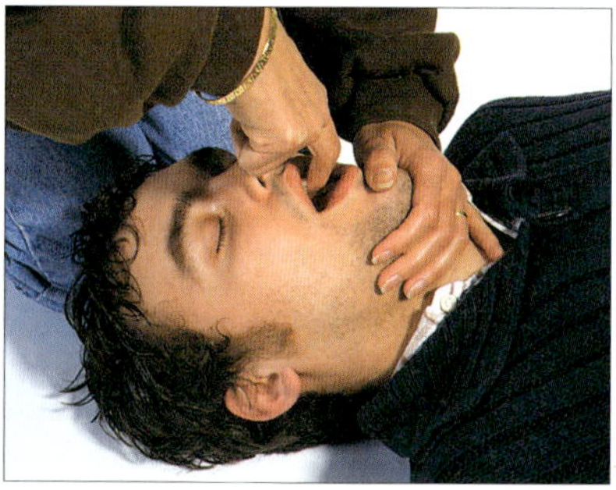

2 With one or two fingers, carefully remove any visible obstructions from the casualty's mouth.

**NEVER** turn the head of a casualty if there is any possibility of a broken or injured neck.

**DO NOT** remove well-fitting dentures that are correctly in place.

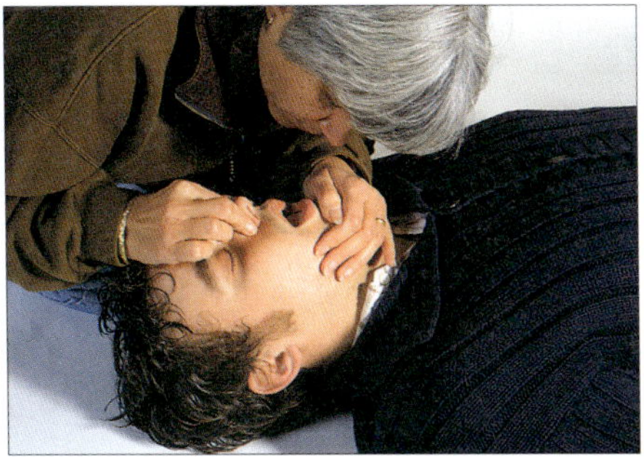

3 If breathing does not commence, give 2 effective rescue breaths (*see page* 26).

4 If the chest does not rise there may still be an obstruction. Recheck the casualty's mouth and recheck that you have tilted the head and lifted the chin adequately. Make up to 5 attempts to achieve 2 effective rescue breaths.

5 If successful, check the circulation (*see page* 22).

6 If you are unable to open the airway and deliver effective rescue breaths, proceed as for choking (*see page* 40).

The throat may close for unknown reasons – for instance, in an allergic attack (*see page* 54) – and it may be impossible to clear the airway. Continue with rescue breathing until help arrives – a little air may make its way to the lungs.

# RESCUE BREATHING

Rescue breathing is one of the most important life-saving procedures you can learn. It is used when the casualty is not breathing.

Rescue breathing is the action of breathing for the casualty by filling his lungs with air.

WHAT TO DO

1 Lay the casualty on his back. Remove any visible obstructions from the mouth. Ensure the airway is clear by tilting the head and lifting the chin.

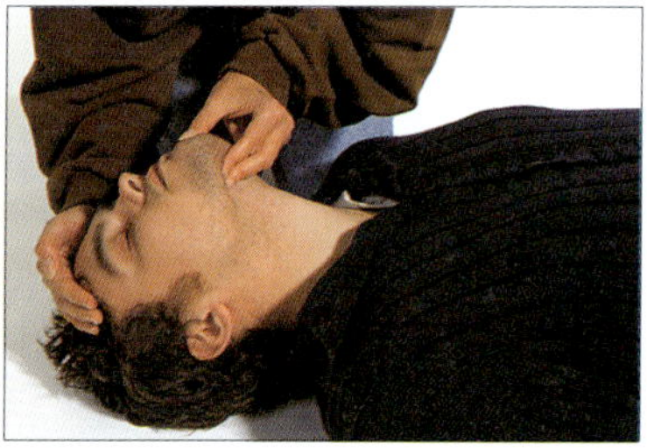

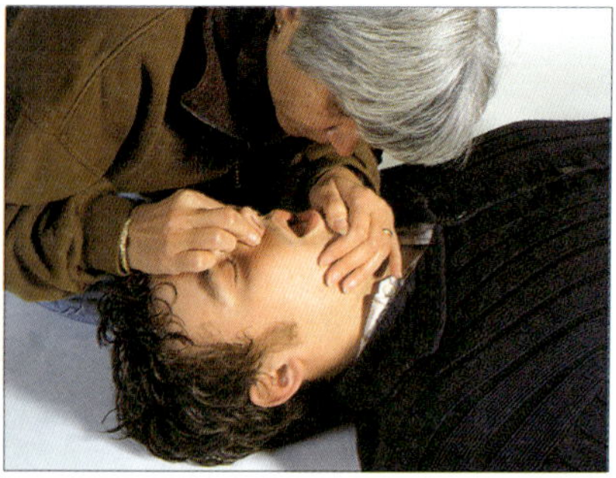

2 Close the casualty's nose by pinching together the nostrils. Take a breath and then place your lips around the casualty's mouth, sealing it so that no air will escape.

3 Breathe into the casualty's mouth for about 1½ –2 seconds until you see the chest rise.

4 Remove your mouth and turn your head to watch the chest fall. Repeat, to give 2 effective rescue breaths in all. If you have difficulty achieving an effective breath, recheck the airway and try again. Make up to 5 attempts in all to achieve 2 effective breaths.

5 **Even if unsuccessful**, move on to assess the circulation (*see page* 22).

6 **If the casualty has a circulation**, continue rescue breathing and recheck for signs of a circulation once a minute.

7 **If the casualty starts to breathe again**, place him in the recovery position (*see page* 34).

8 **If there is no circulation**, or you are unsure, start chest compression (*see page* 29).

MOUTH-TO-NOSE BREATHING

If the casualty has suffered an injury to the mouth, or there is some other reason why mouth-to-mouth resuscitation is impossible, you may need to breathe through the casualty's nose.

1. Close the casualty's mouth firmly and place your mouth around the nose, forming a tight seal.
2. Open the casualty's mouth to allow air to escape as the chest falls, and then cover again while blowing into the nose.

## BABIES AND CHILDREN

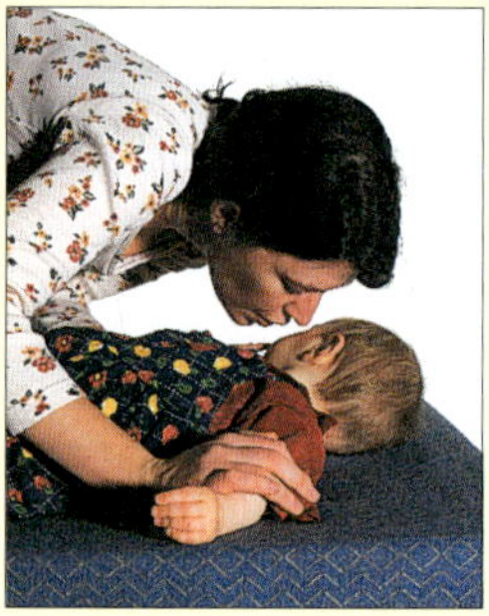

### Babies

When a baby is unconscious and not breathing, resuscitation should be done through the nose and mouth.

1. Tilt the baby's head back and lift the chin to ensure the airway is clear.
2. Seal your lips around the baby's mouth and nose and breathe until you see the chest rise. **Do not** blow too hard.
3. Remove your mouth and allow the chest to fall.
4. Repeat this up to 5 times, giving a minimum of 2 effective breaths.
5. If unsuccessful, recheck the airway and if still unsuccessful, treat for choking (*see page 40*).
6. Assess the circulation (*see page 23*).
7. If the baby has a circulation, continue rescue breathing and recheck for signs of a circulation once a minute.
8. If the baby starts to breathe again, place her in the recovery position (*see page 34*).
9. If there is no circulation, or you are unsure, start chest compression (*see page 31*).

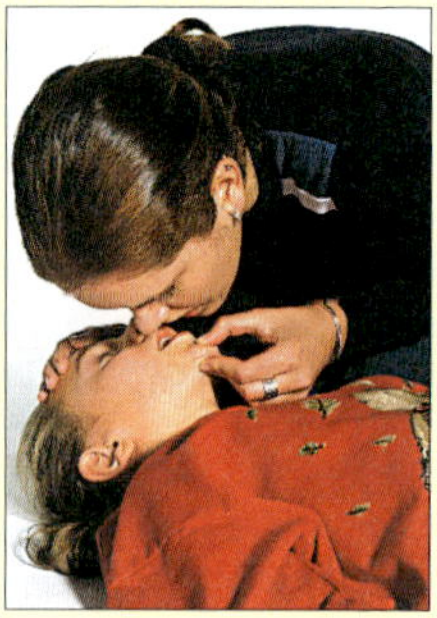

### Children

Children should be ventilated through the mouth, unless there is a mouth injury (*see page 27*). Give up to 5 breaths (a minimum of 2 effective breaths) before assessing the circulation (*see page 23*).

DO NOT blow too hard when resuscitating a baby.

# CHEST COMPRESSION

If there is no circulation after checking for five seconds (*see page 22*), the heart has stopped – the patient has had a 'cardiac arrest' – and you must pump it manually in order for life-giving oxygen to circulate around the body. To ensure that the blood has oxygen in it, always combine chest compression with rescue breathing (*CPR, see page 30*).

NEVER practise chest compression on someone with a beating heart.

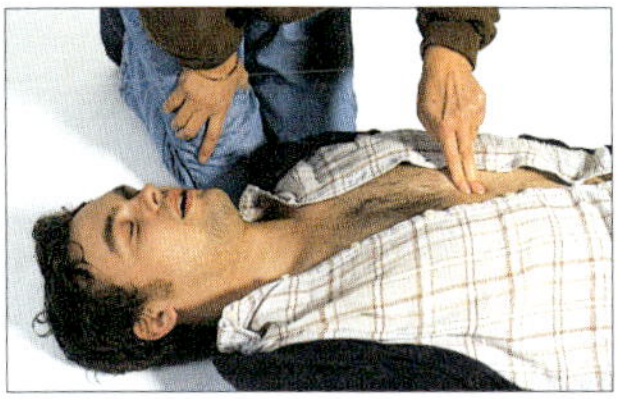

WHAT TO DO

1 Lay him on his back. Find where the lower ribs meet the breastbone and measure 2 finger-widths up from this point.

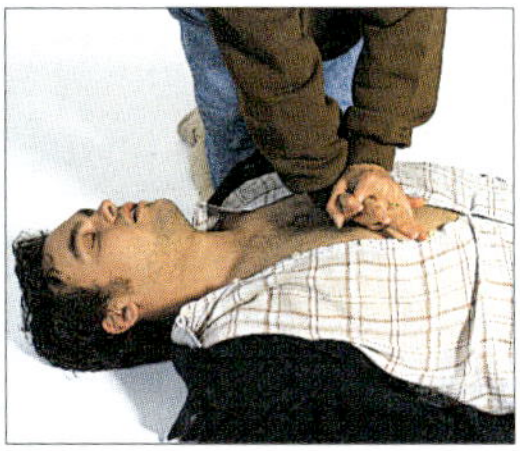

2 Place the heel of your other hand next to the 2 fingers. This is where compression will take place.

3 Place the first hand on top of the other hand and interlock your fingers to keep them away from the casualty's ribs.

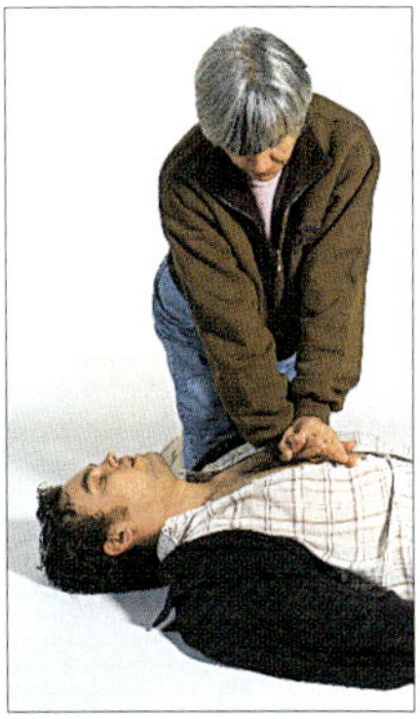

4 With your body centred over the casualty and your arms straight, press down, depressing the chest by about 4–5cm (1½–2in), then release the pressure without removing your hands. Repeat this action at a rate of about 100 per minute. Count out loud to time yourself.

5 Give 15 compressions followed by 2 rescue breaths and continue in cycles of 15:2.

# CARDIOPULMONARY RESUSCITATION (CPR) BY ONE FIRST-AIDER

Cardiopulmonary resuscitation, or CPR, is the combined act of rescue breathing (*see page 26*) and chest compression (*see page 29*).

WHAT TO DO

1 Ensure an ambulance has been called, as soon as you realise the casualty is not breathing (if the casualty has drowned or suffered serious injury, perform resuscitation for a minute before leaving them and making the call, *see page 26*).

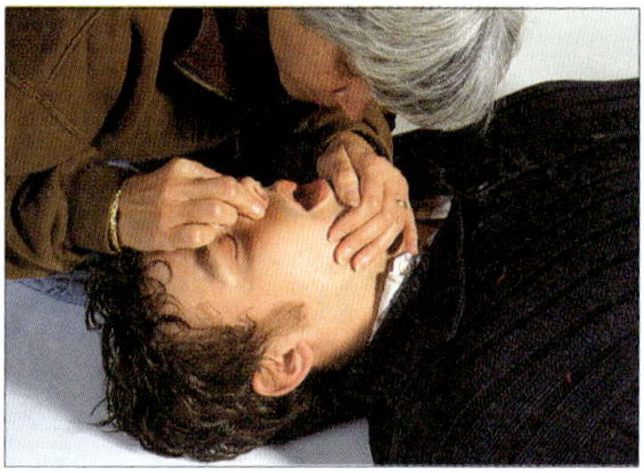

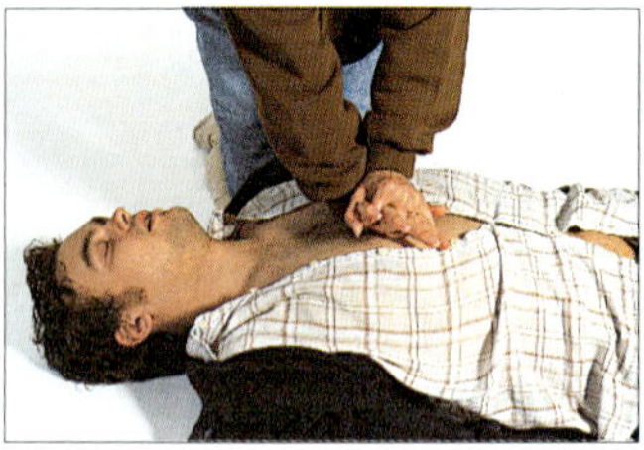

2 Give 2 effective rescue breaths (*see page 26*).

3 Check for a circulation (*see page 22*).

4 If there is no sign of a circulation, or you are unsure, give 15 chest compressions (*see page 29*).

5 Continue in cycles of 2 breaths to 15 chest compressions, until the ambulance arrives.

6 Do not waste time rechecking for breathing or a circulation unless there is an obvious sign of life, e.g. movement or spontaneous breathing.

CPR 'buys time' until the ambulance arrives and professionals try to restart the heart.

## BABIES AND CHILDREN

### Babies

1. If there is no breathing, give up to 5 effective rescue breaths (*see page 28*).

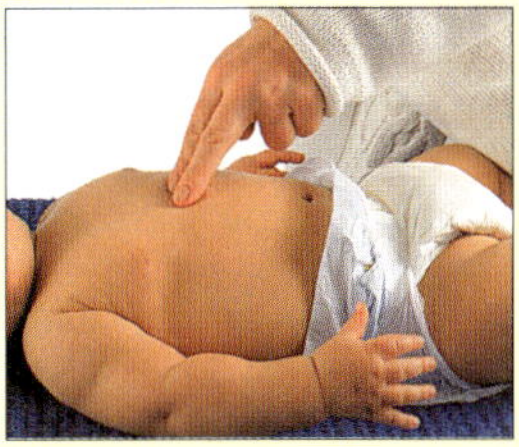

2. Check for a circulation (*see page 23*).
3. If there is no circulation, place the baby on a firm surface and place the tips of two fingers one finger's-width below an imaginary line between the nipples.

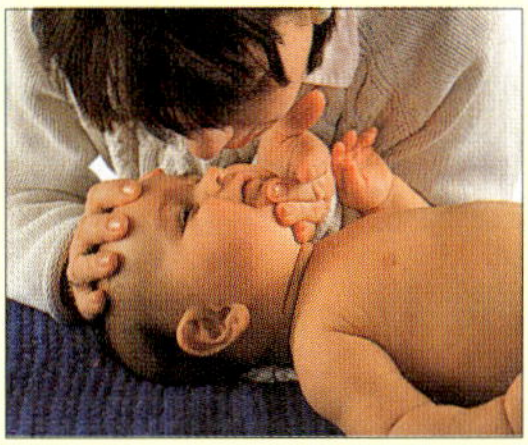

4. Give 5 compressions, pressing at a rate of about 100 compressions per minute. Press hard enough to depress the breastbone about ⅓ of the depth of the baby's chest.

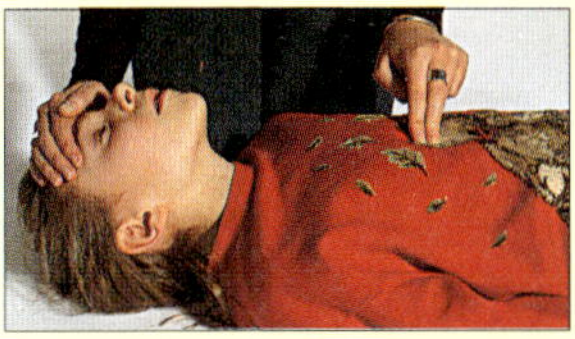

5. Continue in cycles of 1 breath to 5 compressions.
6. If after a minute an ambulance has not already been called, do it yourself, taking the baby with you to the telephone if possible.

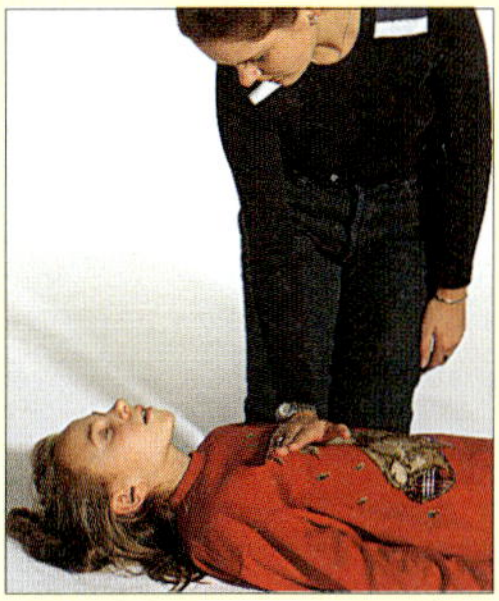

### Children under the Age of 8

1. and 2. *Same as for baby*.
3. If there is no circulation, lay the child on a flat surface and find the point of compression as you would in an adult.
4. Give 5 compressions. Using the heel of one hand only, press at a rate of 100 compressions per minute.
5. and 6. *Same as for baby.*

Children over the age of 8 years should be treated as adults, except that 5 initial rescue breaths are given.

# CARDIOPULMONARY RESUSCITATION (CPR) BY TWO FIRST-AIDERS

Resuscitation can be performed by two first-aiders.

- One breath should be given for every 5 compressions.
- One first-aider will take responsibility for the airway and breathing, while the other compresses the chest.

> DO NOT attempt to breathe into the lungs of the casualty while compression is being performed. One first-aider will deliver one rescue breath for every 5 compressions. The second first-aider will cease compressing while breathing occurs. Count out loud together – 'one, two, three, four, five: blow. One, two, three, four, five: blow'.

WHAT TO DO

1 ☎ One first-aider should kneel by the head of the casualty, taking responsibility for the airway and breathing. If there is no breathing, rescue breathing (*see page 26*) should commence immediately, and an ambulance must be called.

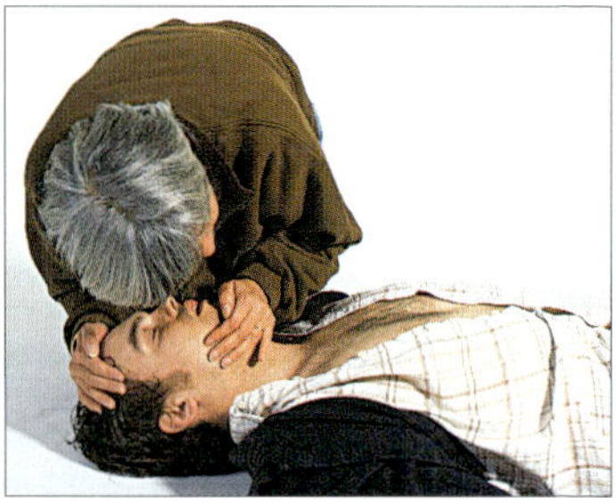

2 Begin with 2 effective rescue breaths.

3 Check for a circulation (*see page* 22). If there is no sign of a circulation, the second first-aider should now begin chest compressions (*see page* 29), pressing down 5 times, and then stopping to allow his companion to give one breath.

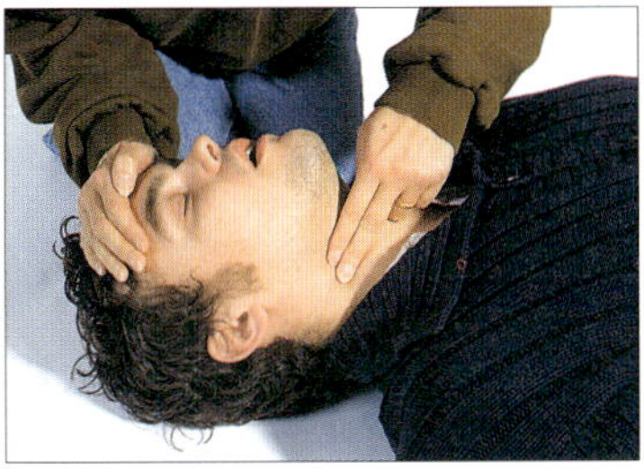

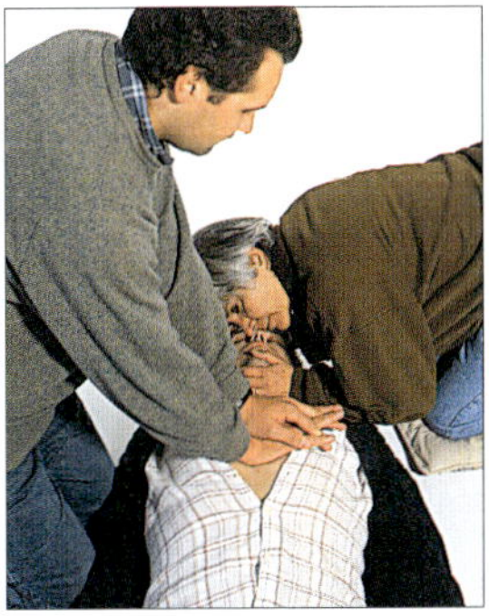

4 Give 1 breath for every 5 compressions, and repeat until help arrives. Do not waste time checking the breathing or for a circulation unless there is an obvious sign of life, e.g. movement or spontaneous breathing.

5 If the first-aider performing chest compressions becomes tired, the roles should be reversed.

# RECOVERY POSITION

The recovery position is probably the most important position used in an emergency situation. When a casualty who is unconscious, semi-conscious, or in danger of becoming unconscious is left on her back, there are a number of dangerous situations which can arise, including:

- The tongue falling back and blocking the airway.
- Blood, vomit, water or other substances entering the airway because the opening to the larynx does not close upon contact (its normal response).

The recovery position allows the tongue to fall forward so that the airway remains clear from obstruction and any foreign substances, such as blood or vomit, can drain away.

ALWAYS take extreme care when moving somebody with a suspected neck injury.

Before placing the casualty in the recovery position, follow the ABC of resuscitation (*see page 21*). If the casualty is unconscious and is breathing you should put them in the recovery position.

Remove the casualty's spectacles and check that pockets are empty – keys, etc can be very painful and cause significant damage to tissues if a casualty is left to lie on them for only a few minutes.

## WHAT TO DO

1 Kneel beside the casualty, and open the airway (tilt the head back and lift the chin, *see page 21*).

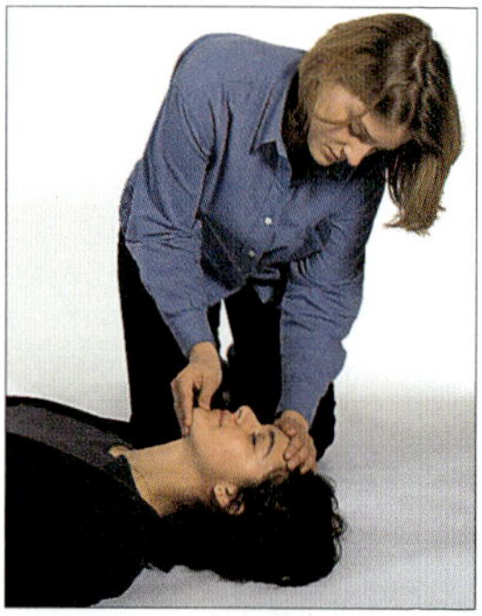

2 Straighten the casualty's legs and then tuck the arm nearest to you, arm straight and palm upwards, under the thigh.

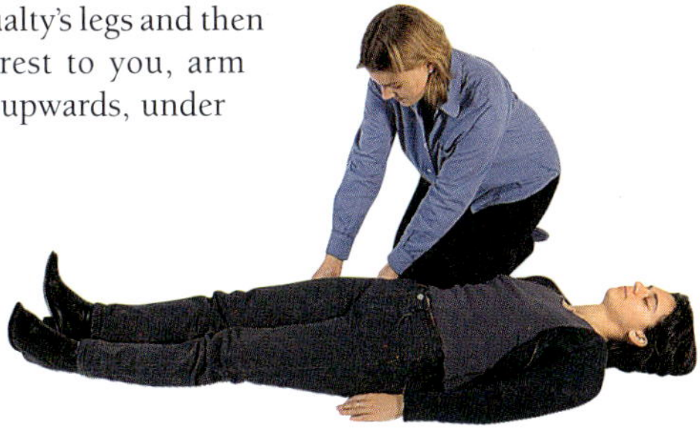

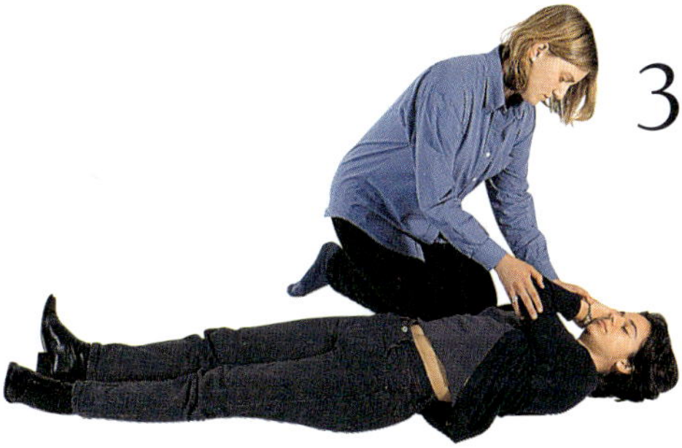

3 Take the other arm across the body and hold the back of the hand against the casualty's cheek.

4 Bend the knee furthest from you, keeping the casualty's foot on the ground.

5 Keep the hand pressed against the cheek and pull on the bent knee to roll the casualty towards you, ensuring the head is supported. Adjust the upper leg so that hip and knee are both bent at right angles. Adjust lower arm so that the casualty is not lying on it.

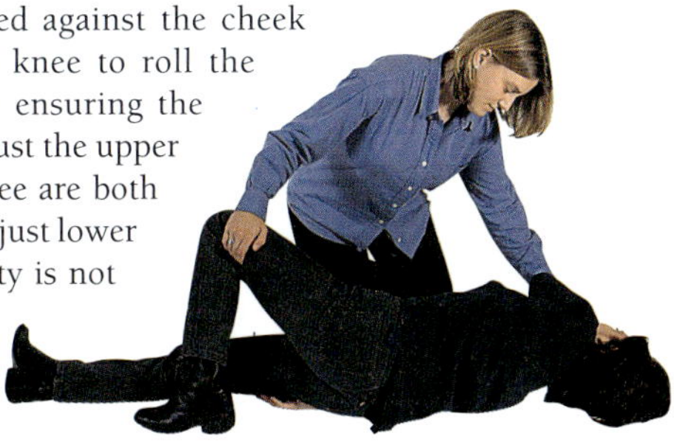

6 Tilt the head back to ensure the airway is clear (*see page 21*); adjust the hand under the cheek, if necessary, to keep head tilted.

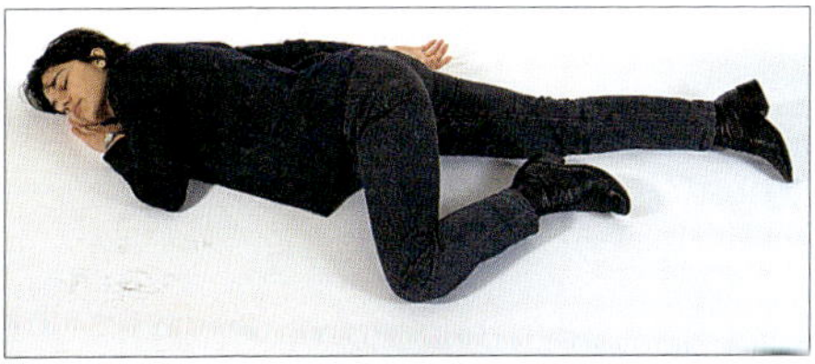

7 Continue to check breathing regularly. Do not leave the casualty unattended, if possible, and ensure an ambulance is called.

# TREATING AN UNCONSCIOUS CASUALTY

Unconsciousness occurs when the casualty's normal brain function is interrupted. In this condition, normal reflexes may not work.

> NEVER give an unconscious casualty anything to eat or drink.

To assess whether a casualty is unconscious or simply sleeping:
- Gently shake her shoulders.
- Shout in her ear.

There are many causes of unconsciousness, and you should, as soon as you realise the casualty is in this condition, follow the ABC of resuscitation (*see page 21*) and then try to ascertain why. Check for needle marks, which may mean injections of insulin or drugs. Look for signs of alcohol or drug abuse. Look for medical warning signs such as a Medic Alert bracelet or necklace (which will give the condition the casualty suffers from), or a card indicating that the casualty suffers from a condition such as epilepsy or diabetes.

Other causes of unconsciousness include:
- Head injury (*see page 94*).
- Stroke (*see page 112*).
- Conditions in which oxygen cannot enter the bloodstream – perhaps an obstruction in the airway, or an injury which causes damage to the lungs.
- Diabetes (*see page 77*) and epilepsy (*see page 72*).

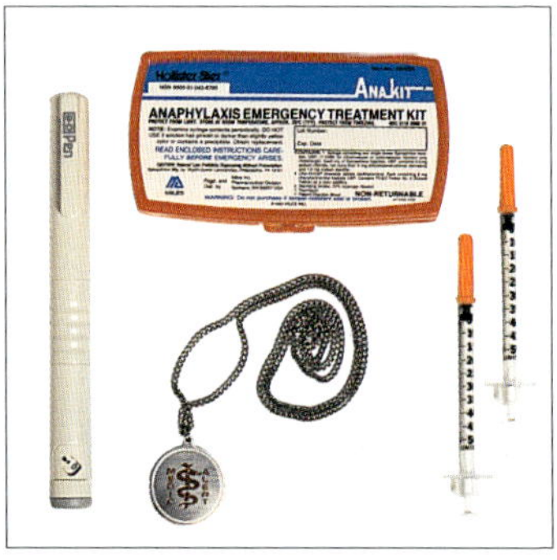


*Right*: Signs that a casualty suffers from a medical condition. *Clockwise from the top*: Anaphylaxis emergency treatment kit (for treating severe allergic reactions); diabetic insulin 'pen'; insulin needles; *Centre*: Medic Alert necklace (similar bracelets are also found).

Any information you have ascertained about the casualty's condition should be passed on to the emergency medical services as soon as possible, to allow them to prepare for treatment.

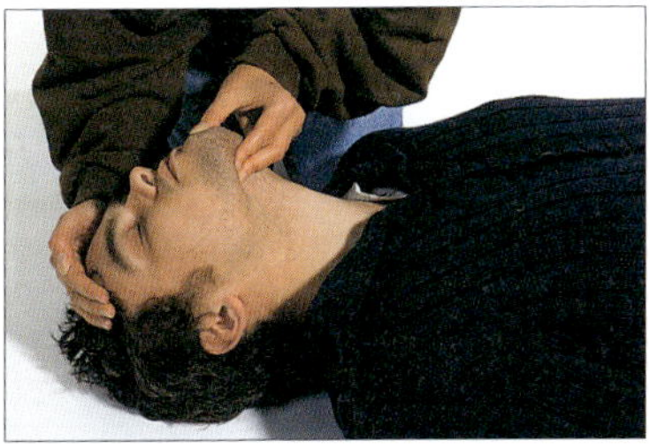

WHAT TO DO

1 Follow the ABC of Resuscitation (*see page 21*).

**If breathing**

1 Place him in the recovery position (*see page 34*) and check his breathing regularly.

2 ☎ Call for an ambulance.

**If not breathing but with a circulation**

1 ☎ Call for an ambulance.

2 Perform rescue breathing (*see page 26*).

3 Check for a circulation about every minute.

4 If breathing returns, place him in the recovery position (*see page 34*).

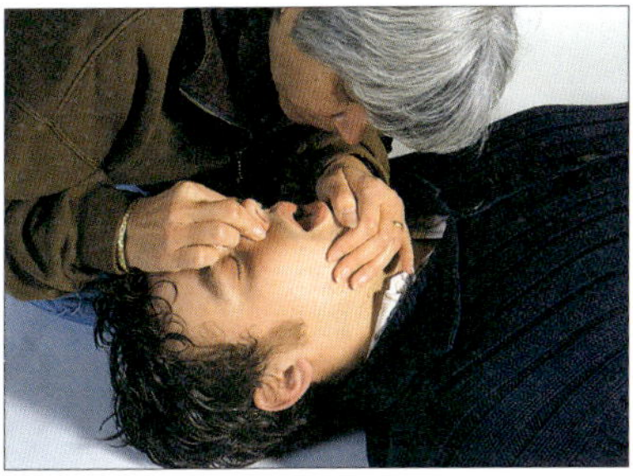

**If not breathing, with no pulse**

1 ☎ Call for an ambulance immediately.

2 Perform rescue breathing together with chest compressions (CPR, *see page 30*).

If possible, DO NOT tilt the head to clear the airway of a casualty who may have a broken or injured neck. Only lift the chin.

BABIES

1. Attempt to rouse the baby by gently pinching or prodding her. Do not shake the baby.
2. Shout for help.
3. Tilt her head back slightly and lift the chin to open the airway (*see page 24* if blocked).

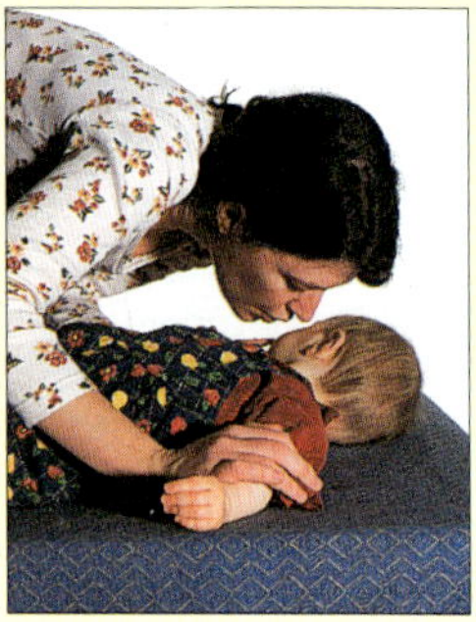

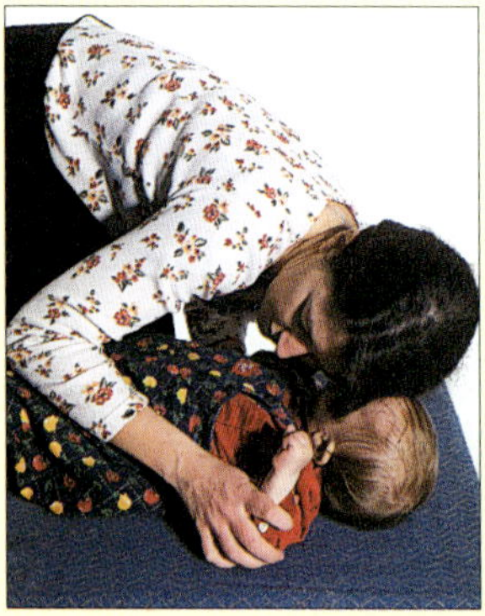

4. ☎ Look, listen and feel for breathing. If the casualty is breathing, place her in the recovery position (*see page 34*) and call for an ambulance.
5. If there is no breathing give 5 rescue breaths (*see page 28*).
6. ☎ Check circulation. If there is a circulation, continue rescue breathing and call for an ambulance.
7. ☎ If there is no circulation, give 5 chest compressions and call for an ambulance.
8. Continue CPR (*see page 31*) if necessary, until ambulance arrives.

DO NOT blow too hard when resuscitating a baby.

CHILDREN

1. Attempt to rouse the child, gently pinching or prodding her and shouting.
2. Shout for help.

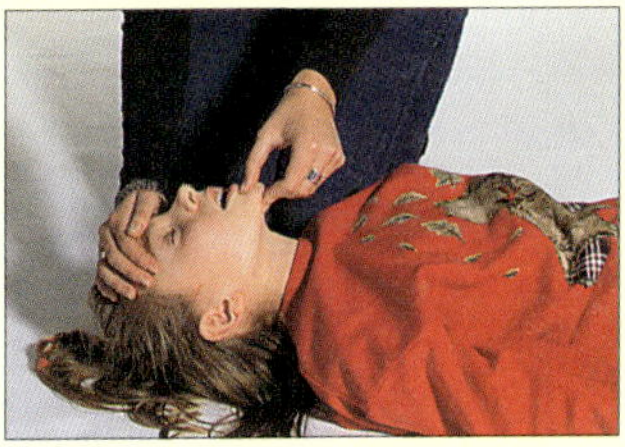

3. Open the airway (*see page 24* if blocked).

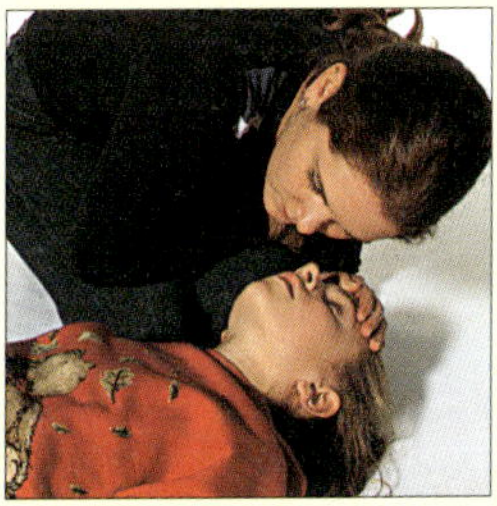

4. ☎ Look, listen and feel for breathing (*see page 22*). If the casualty is breathing, place her in the recovery position (*see page 34*) and call for an ambulance.
5. If there is no breathing give 5 rescue breaths (*see page 28*).
6. ☎ Check circulation. If there is a circulation, continue rescue breathing and call for an ambulance.
7. ☎ If there is no circulation, give 5 chest compressions and call for an ambulance.
8. Continue CPR (*see page 31*) if necessary, until ambulance arrives.

# TREATMENT OF CHOKING

When a casualty is choking it is essential that every effort is made to remove the obstruction by coughing, back blows or the abdominal thrust (Heimlich Manoeuvre).

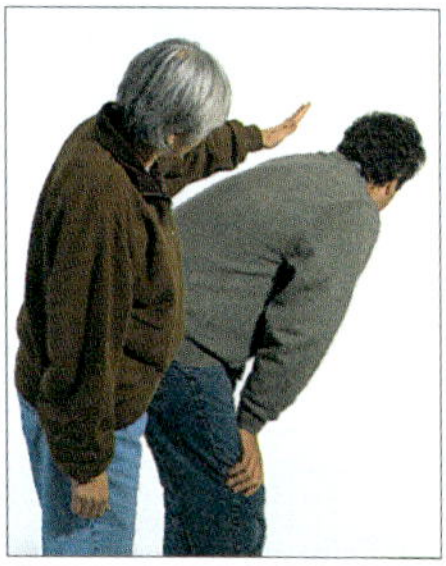

## BACK BLOWS

Before intervening in any way, encourage the casualty to cough vigorously if possible. If unable to clear the obstruction proceed to give 5 hard blows to the back between the shoulder blades with the flat of the hand. If unsuccessful, procede to abdominal thrusts. Alternate 5 back blows and 5 abdominal thrusts until the obstruction is relieved.

## THE ABDOMINAL THRUST (HEIMLICH MANOEUVRE)

The abdominal thrust is used when other attempts to dislodge an obstruction in the airway of a casualty fail. It can be used on both conscious and unconscious victims of choking. This manoeuvre works by driving a sudden burst of air from the lungs, which should expel anything blocking the airway.

### If conscious

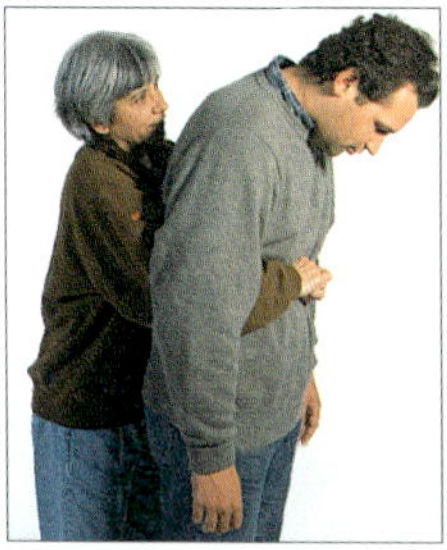

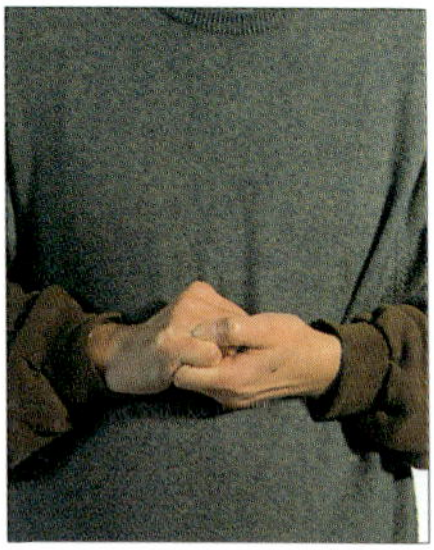

WHAT TO DO

1 Stand behind the casualty and place your arm around him, under his ribcage.

2 Join your hands together just below the bottom of the breastbone and pull one fist in with the other hand in a short, sharp thrust inwards and upwards.

3 Repeat this procedure up to 5 times if the obstruction is not freed.

4 Alternate 5 back blows with 5 abdominal thrusts until the obstruction is relieved, checking to see if the airway is open with rescue breaths after each cycle.

## If unconscious

### WHAT TO DO

1 Kneel over the casualty and place the heel of your hand just below the bottom of the breastbone.

2 With your other hand on top, press inwards and upwards in a short, sharp thrust. This is an abdominal thrust.

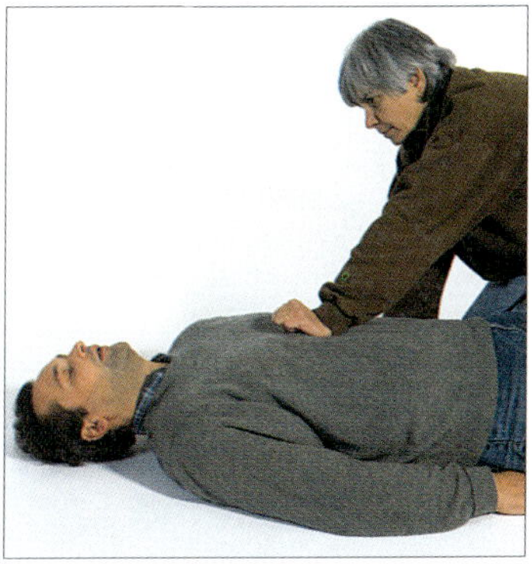

3 Repeat this procedure if the obstruction is not freed.

4 Alternate 5 back blows with 5 abdominal thrusts until the obstruction is cleared, checking to see if the airway is open with rescue breaths after each cycle.

(*see also Choking, page 68*)

### BABIES (LESS THAN 1 YEAR)

- NEVER use abdominal thrusts on a baby.
- Alternate 5 back blows with 5 chest thrusts until the obstruction is relieved, checking to see if the airway is open with rescue breaths after each cycle.

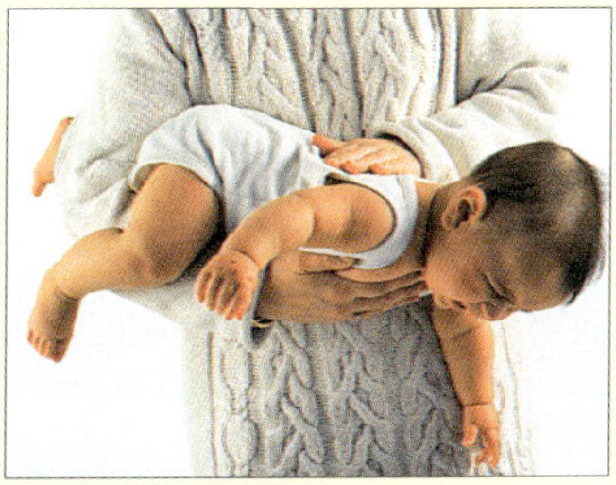

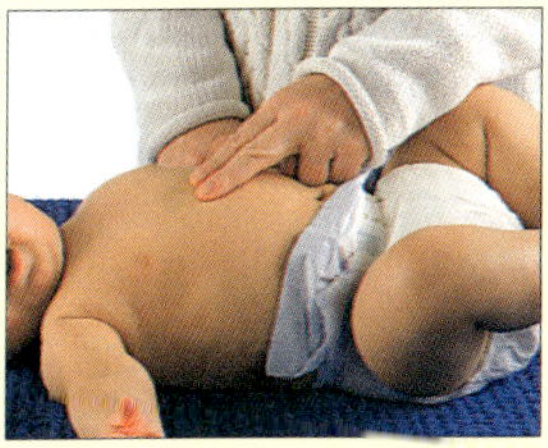

The technique for chest thrusts is similar to that for chest compressions (*see page* 29), but they are performed with a sharper, more vigorous action, at a rate of about 20 a minute.

**Children**

A child who is choking may be able to confirm this, and she may be able to cough to eject the obstruction. If this does not work, follow these steps.

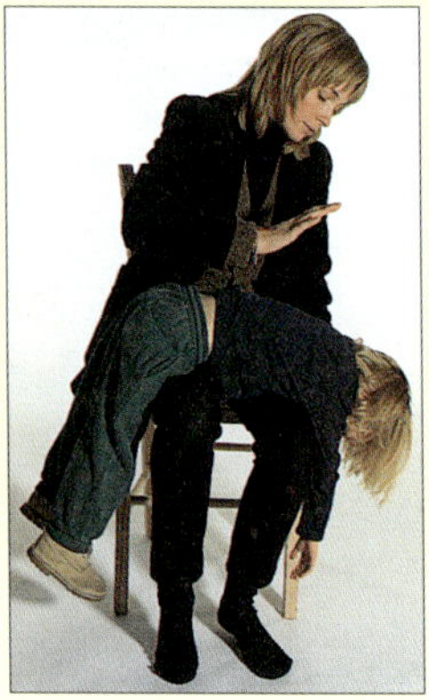

1. Lay a small child across your lap face down and deliver up to 5 back blows between the shoulder blades.
2. If the blows fail, perform up to 5 chest thrusts using a similar technique to chest compressions (*see page 29*) but a sharper, more vigorous action, and at a rate of about 20 per minute.

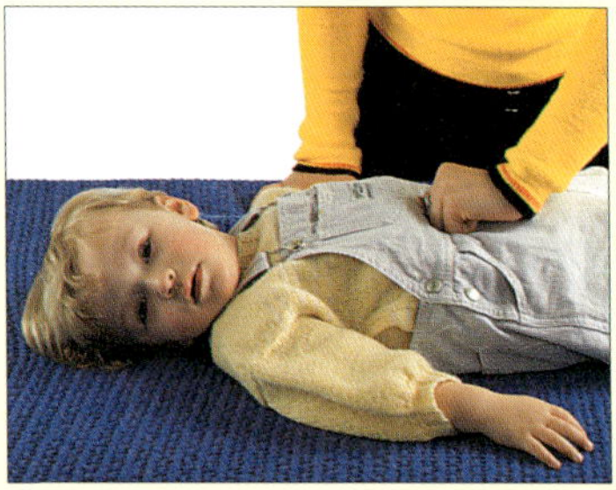

3. If these fail, give 5 more back blows followed by 5 abdominal thrusts, using just one hand.
4. Alternate back blows with abdominal or chest thrusts in subsequent cycles. Check to see if the airway is open with rescue breaths after each cycle.

NEVER perform blind finger sweeps of the mouth as these may cause further damage. If the child does not breathe after 5 back blows and 5 chest thrusts, attempt to give 5 rescue breaths (*see page 28*). Check to see if the airway has cleared with rescue breaths after each cycle.

Act quickly. Starving the body of oxygen causes brain damage and eventually death. Call for help if you have any trouble clearing the throat, and continue treatment until it arrives.

# CONTROLLING BLEEDING

Bleeding occurs when an injury causes blood to be lost from the blood vessels. There are two types:

- Internal bleeding occurs when blood escapes from the circulatory system, but not from the body itself. This is called a closed wound – e.g. broken bone, ruptured spleen.
- External bleeding occurs when blood escapes from the circulatory system via an opening in the skin. This is called an open wound.

Bleeding is potentially very dangerous, because a severe loss of blood can lead to shock (*see page 46*). Infection is also able to enter the body through the wound.

> Remember there may be a risk of cross-infection. Cover any of your own sores or wounds with a plaster before administering treatment to someone who is bleeding. If possible, wear disposable gloves. Wash your hands carefully with soap and hot water before and after treatment.

The priorities of resuscitation will remain the same, no matter how alarming the bleeding may appear.

> Remember the ABC of resuscitation (*see page 21*). Very occasionally the airway may be blocked by bleeding which will have to be stopped. But in most cases, bleeding should be dealt with after you have cleared the airway, ensured that the casualty is breathing and that there is a circulation.

Emergency treatment of external wounds is aimed at controlling the bleeding and preventing the onset of shock (*see page 46*). If you suspect internal bleeding, you must get the casualty to hospital as soon as possible.

# External Bleeding

WHAT TO DO

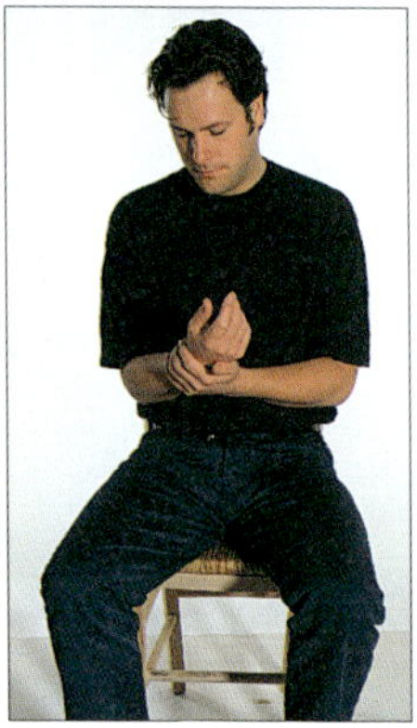

1 Remove casualty's clothing (*see page 156*). Don't try to remove any objects in the wound and be careful that you do not wound yourself trying to perform treatment.

2 Squeeze the sides of the wound together; apply direct pressure to the wound with your fingers, hand or preferably a pad made from a clean bandage or from a handkerchief. An article of clean clothing will do.

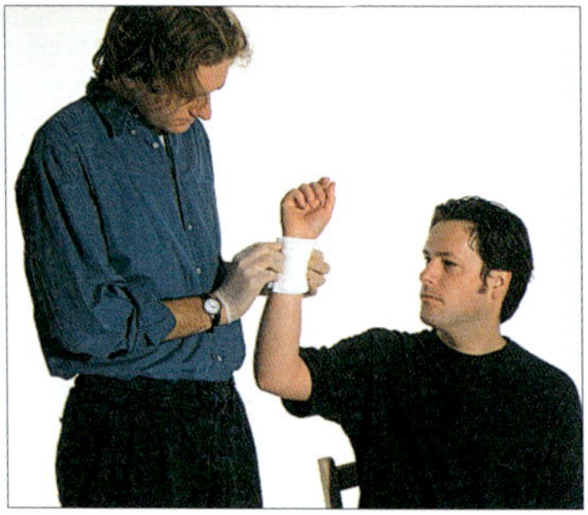

3 An injured limb should be raised and supported above the level of the heart. This may be easiest if the casualty is lying down.

DO NOT move a casualty if there is a risk of fracture to the head, neck or spine.

4 Firmly bandage the original pad in place, but take care not to cut off the circulation to the area. If there is an object still protruding from the wound, pad either side until a bandage can be wrapped around it without pressing it further into the wound.

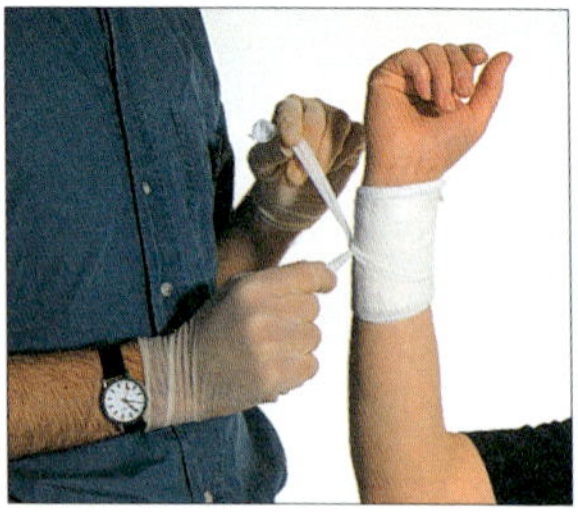

5 Watch carefully for signs of shock.

6 ☎ Call for an ambulance.

## *Internal Bleeding*

☎ If you suspect that an injury may have caused internal bleeding, the most important steps are to prevent shock from occurring. Urgent medical attention is necessary, so call for an ambulance as soon as possible.

Signs of internal bleeding include:
- Cold, clammy white or grey skin.
- A weak, rapid pulse.
- Pain in the injured area.
- Intense thirst and confusion.

1 With extreme care, lay the casualty down and raise his feet to a level above his head. Use folded blankets or clothing, a car tyre or books.

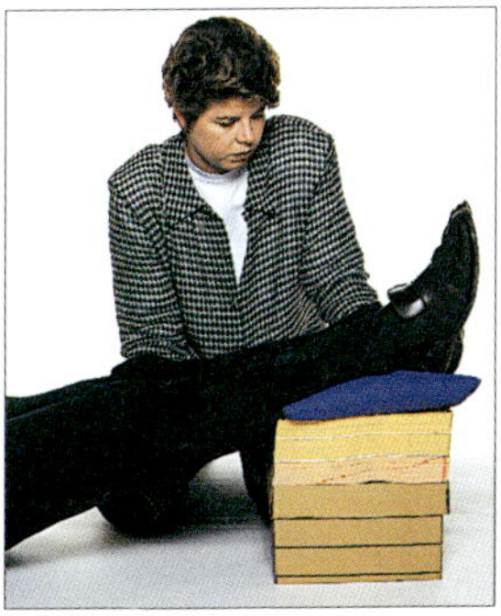

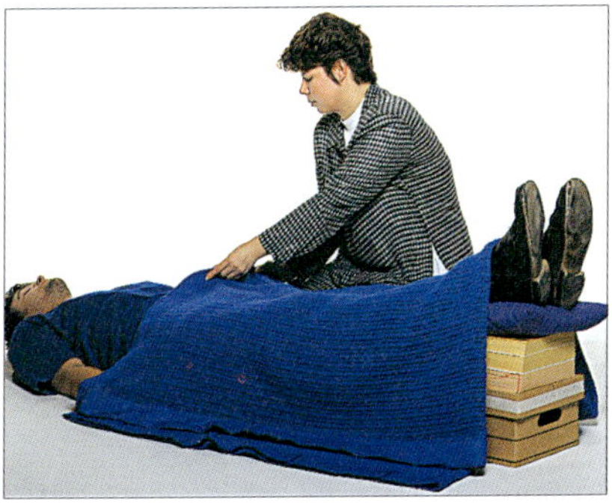

2 ☎ Call for an ambulance immediately and advise the emergency services of the type of injury (if known).

3 Follow the ABC of resuscitation (*see page 21*).

> If at any stage the casualty becomes unconscious or begins to vomit, place him in the recovery position (*see page 34*).

(*See also Bleeding and Wounds, page 58, Dressings, page 132, and Bandages, page 135*).

# TREATING SHOCK

In modern-day English, the word shock has come to mean 'fright', which has nothing to do with the meaning of the clinical term. Clinical shock means a profound fall in blood pressure. This may be the result of blood loss (*see page 93*), loss of tissue fluid (*see Burns, page 49*) or heart failure (*see page 66*). It means that the fluid in the blood vessels is of an insufficient quantity to carry oxygenated blood around the body, to the heart, lungs, brain and other essential organs. When the pumping action of the heart is inadequate to carry blood throughout the body, the body goes into a state of clinical shock and it begins to shut down arteries which serve less important parts of the body, like the skin or the digestive system. However, if the shock remains untreated, the body will eventually shut down altogether – a fatal condition.

There are many causes for shock, including:

- Heart failure – the heart is unable to pump the blood around the body.
- Haemorrhaging – blood loss means that there is insufficient blood in the blood vessels to maintain blood pressure, which drops, preventing the essential flow of oxygenated blood to the organs.
- Burns – serious burns cause a loss of fluid, which causes dehydration and a decrease in the blood volume.
- Infections – serious infections, such as septicaemia (an infection of the blood itself) may force the blood vessels to widen, leaking fluid from the blood into the tissues. This causes a shortage of blood in the vessels and a drop in blood pressure.
- Dehydration – caused by vomiting or diarrhoea, which draws fluid from the blood and leads to a decrease in volume.
- Anaphylaxis (*see Allergic Attack, page 54*)

NEVER give a casualty with shock anything to eat or drink, no matter how thirsty he appears. The casualty must not attempt to smoke.

## *Signs of Shock*

As shock sets in, there is an initial rush of adrenaline as the body struggles to maintain blood pressure. Less important functions are then shut down in an attempt to redistribute the circulation. The following symptoms will occur as shock develops:

- Rapid, weak pulse.

- Cold sweat, causing the skin to feel clammy.
- Pale, grey skin and occasionally blueness around the mouth.
- Weakness.
- Nausea and occasionally vomiting.
- Extreme thirst and overwhelming fatigue, causing the casualty to yawn. Confusion, agitation and aggression can also be a feature.
- Severe breathlessness.
- Possible loss of consciousness when the blood supply to the brain is insufficient because of the fall in blood pressure.

NEVER leave a casualty with shock alone and reassure him constantly. Panic will make the condition much worse.

☎ First-aiders must attempt to halt the course of shock and allow the body to best distribute the circulation. Call for an ambulance as soon as you suspect shock – or ask someone else to do so.

WHAT TO DO

1 Lay the casualty down and raise her feet above the level of her head – on some folded blankets or clothing, a car tyre or some books. This encourages the flow of blood to the major organs instead of to the legs.

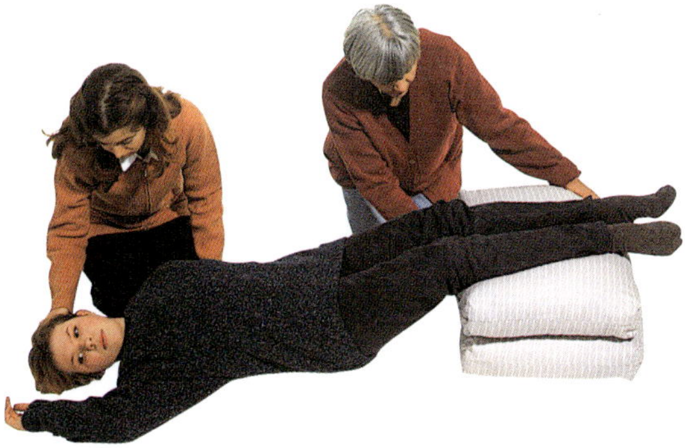

2 Treat any obvious wounds (*see page 58*).

3 Loosen any tight clothing and ensure that the casualty does not move.

4 Cover the body with a single coat or blanket – never allow a victim of shock to overheat or get too cold.

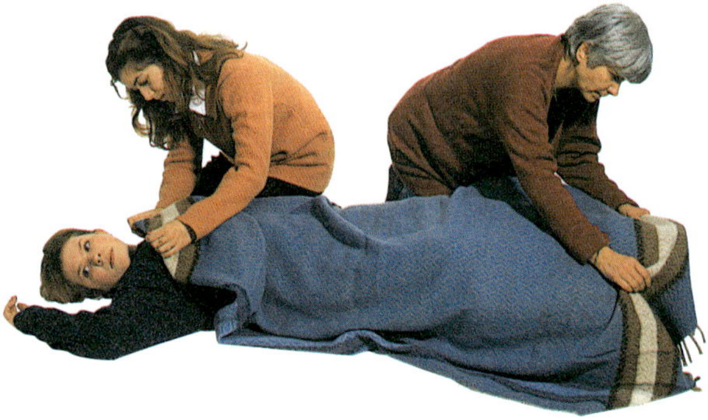

5 Continue to check circulation and breathing every 2–3 minutes.

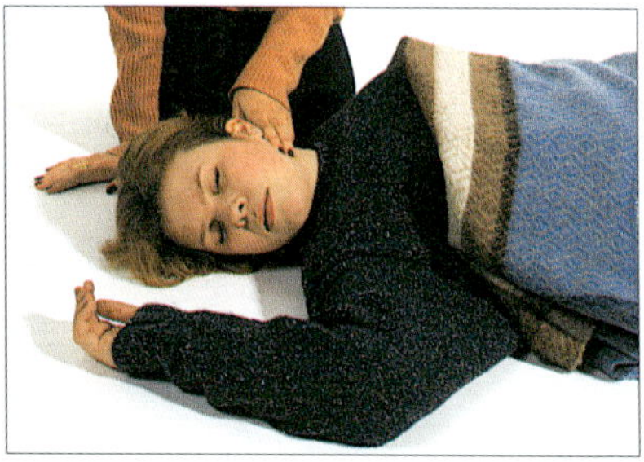

If the victim's breathing or circulation stops at any point, begin rescue breathing or CPR immediately (*see pages 26, 30*).

If there is any chance of fracture or neck or back injury, do not move the casualty unless the situation is dangerous.

The legs should be raised and supported immediately, but you should take a few moments to stabilise an injury (*see page 86*) if movement could make it worse.

If breathing becomes difficult or if there is vomiting, place the casualty in the recovery position (*see page 34*) and follow the ABC of resuscitation (*see page 21*).

# TREATING BURNS

A burn is an injury to the skin and tissue caused by extreme heat or cold, by radiation (including sunlight), corrosive substances, electricity and friction. Scalds are burns which are the result of wet heat, like hot water or steam vapours. There are three types of burn, of varying severity:

- **Superficial**, where the surface layer of the skin is burnt, resulting in redness and some swelling and tenderness. Superficial burns do not usually require medical attention, but they must be kept clean and dry to avoid infection.
- **Partial thickness**, where deeper parts of the skin are damaged. Partial thickness burns normally blister and are at risk of infection. They should be seen by a doctor, but normally heal well.

Anyone with partial or superficial burns covering more than 9 per cent of the body should seek immediate medical attention. As a rough guide look at the palm of the hand of the casualty (palm of hand = 1 per cent of body surface).

- **Deep**, or full-thickness, where all layers of the skin are burnt, appearing grey, waxy and occasionally charred. Deep burns may often be painless due to nerve damage. All deep burns must receive urgent medical attention.

Burns on the face and over joints should be medically assessed, no matter what the size.

(*See also Burns and Scalds, page 62*).

The main priorities when treating burn victims are to:

- Ensure your own safety.
- Remove the casualty from risk of further burning.
- Provide resuscitation if necessary.
- Provide rapid cooling.
- ☎ Call for an ambulance, explaining the type of burn (if known) and giving other information which may help (extent of burns, position, age of casualty and any other relevant details).
- Treat for shock or other injuries.
- Prevent risk of infection.

ABC of resuscitation is the priority (*see page 21*). If possible, get someone else to do the cooling while you follow the procedure.

## *Serious Burns and Scalds*

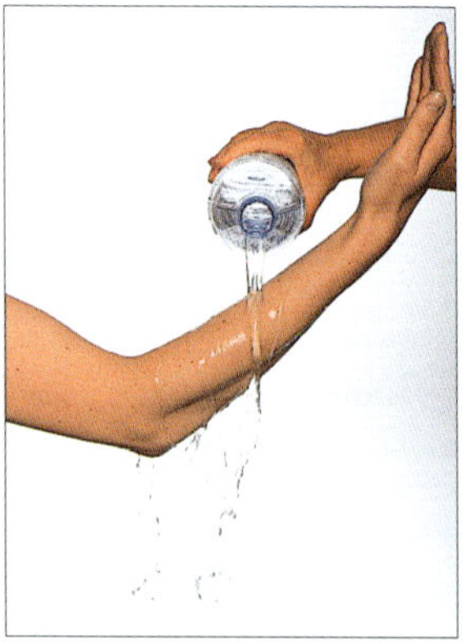

WHAT TO DO

The ABC of resuscitation is the main priority if required (*see page 21*).

1 Unless there is a risk of fracture or other injury to the neck, head or back, lay the casualty on his back and pour cold water on the burned area.

2 ☎ Call for an ambulance and resume pouring cold water on the burned area. It may take upwards of 10 minutes to cool the burn.

3 While cooling the burns, follow the ABC of resuscitation if required (*see page 21*). If the casualty needs to be resuscitated, try to get help so that the cooling can continue while resuscitating (*see page 26*).

4 Remove clothing around the burn. Never remove anything that seems to be stuck to the burn as this can cause further damage and lead to infection. Cut around clothing if necessary (*see page 156*).

If cold running water is unavailable, use any cold substance that will not cause further injury, such as milk, fruit juice or tinned drinks.

5 Cover the injury with a clean, preferably sterile bandage that is not fluffy. Cotton-wool is not appropriate. Use a burns sheet or a clean sheet. In an emergency, cover loosely with cling film, several lengths in from the beginning of the roll.

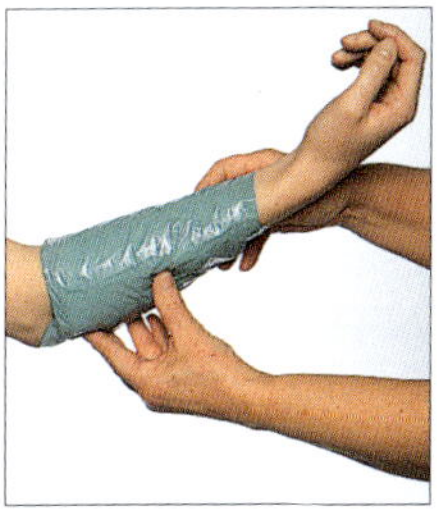

BURNS SHEET

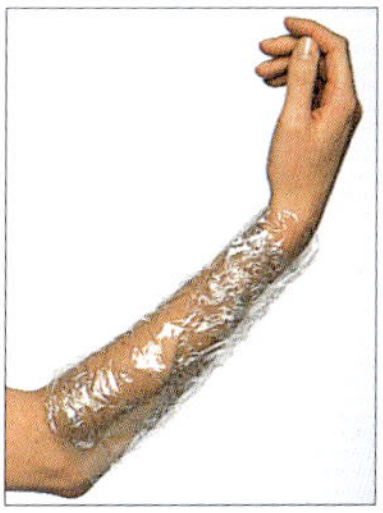

CLING FILM

NEVER wrap cling film tightly around a limb. The limb cannot swell and the circulation may become impaired.

Only use cling film when the burn is cool – otherwise it will stick to the skin.

6 Treat the casualty for shock (*see page 46*) while waiting for medical help and check breathing and circulation every 3–4 minutes until help arrives. Be prepared to begin rescue breathing and CPR (*see pages 26, 30*) in the event that breathing or circulation stops.

- DO NOT touch or pat at the injured area.
- Always pour water over the burned area, never use a compress or cloth.
- DO NOT apply ointment, butter, lotions or antiseptics.
- DO NOT burst blisters as they protect from infection.
- DO NOT overcool the casualty as this can lead to shock or hypothermia.

## *Burns to the Mouth and Throat*

Any burns to the airway should be treated urgently at a hospital. With all burns there is a serious risk of swelling and inflammation, and in the throat or mouth this can cut off the essential supply of oxygen.

You will recognise burns to this area by:

- Indication of burning to the area (charring, singeing of the nostril hairs, burnt tongue or blistering around the mouth).
- Pain in the mouth and throat area.

- Breathing difficulties.
- Shock (*see page* 46).
- If you see soot around the mouth/nose you should be very vigilant as burns to airway may be present.

WHAT TO DO

1 ☎ Before any treatment is considered, call for an ambulance. Specialist medical attention is required urgently.

2 Loosen clothing from around the neck area.

3 Follow the ABC of resuscitation. **If the casualty is unconscious and breathing**, place her in the recovery position (*see page* 34) and check breathing regularly (*see page* 22). Resuscitation may be necessary, so be prepared (*see page* 26).

# EMERGENCY CONDITIONS

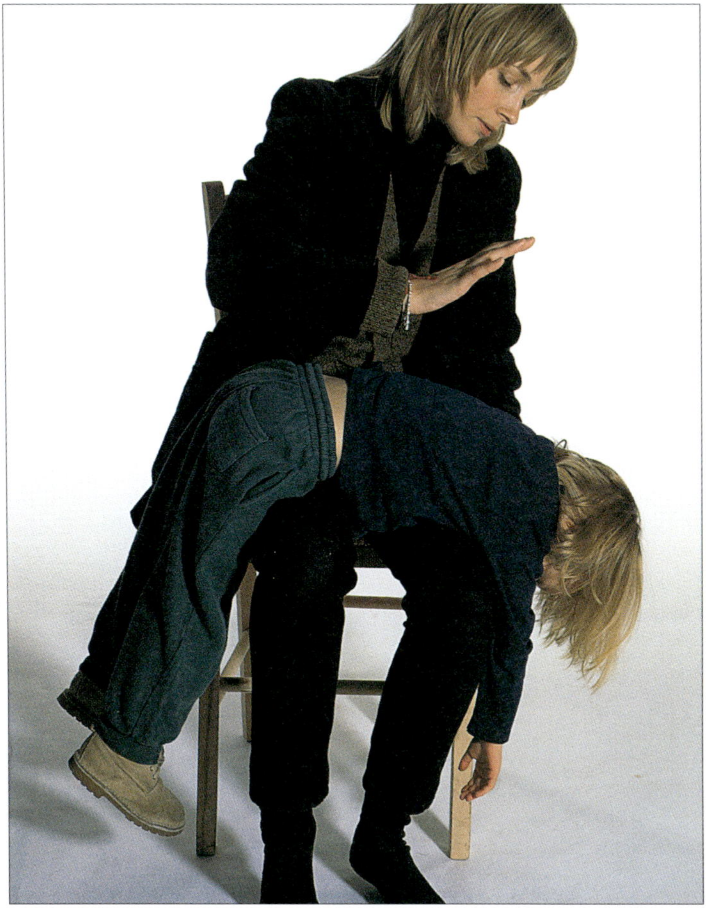

# ALLERGIC ATTACK

Allergies are a hostile reaction by the body to substances that are normally considered to be harmless. For some reason, the body looks upon these substances – for example, pollens, foods, drugs, pets, house dust mites, chemicals and others – as an invader, and antibodies are produced to defend the body against them. In less severe cases, this reaction may manifest itself as hives, itching, running eyes; food allergies may produce vomiting, abdominal pain or cramps and diarrhoea. Hay fever is an example of an allergic reaction with annoying but not life-threatening symptoms. Very severe allergy can produce a reaction called anaphylactic shock, which is a very serious, acute allergic reaction that may cause death unless treated immediately. Some of the most common causes of this massive allergic reaction in sensitive people are:

- Insect stings; for instance, bees or wasps.
- Ingestion of a food substance, e.g. milk, eggs, sesame seeds, or peanuts.
- Injection or ingestion of drugs such as penicillin.

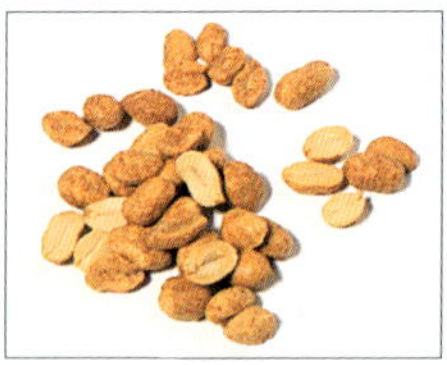

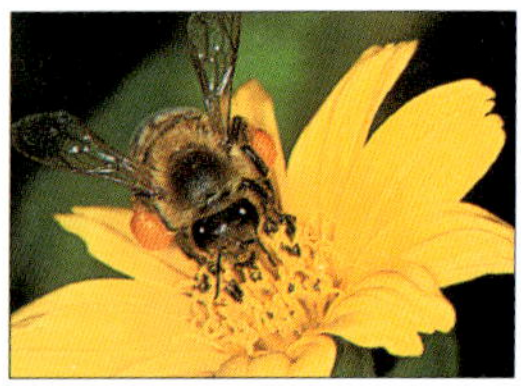

Symptoms of this type of shock include:

- Swelling of the lips, tongue and face.
- Shortness of breath, wheezing, asthma and a croaky voice.
- Sudden violent rash.
- Vomiting, diarrhoea and abdominal pain.
- Falling blood pressure, dizziness and loss of consciousness.

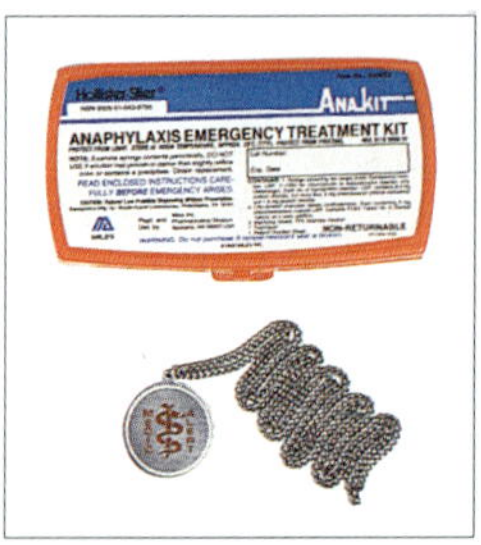


Unless the casualty receives oxygen and an injection of adrenaline, he may die. Your first priority will always be to get him to hospital.

*Left:* Signs that a casualty suffers from an allergic condition: *top*: Anaphylaxis emergency kit; *bottom*: Medic Alert necklace (similar bracelets are also found), these give the condition the casualty suffers from.

WHAT TO DO

1 ☎ Call for an ambulance and provide as much information as you can about what may be causing the reaction. Make it clear to the emergency services that anaphylaxis is occurring – not all ambulances carry adrenaline.

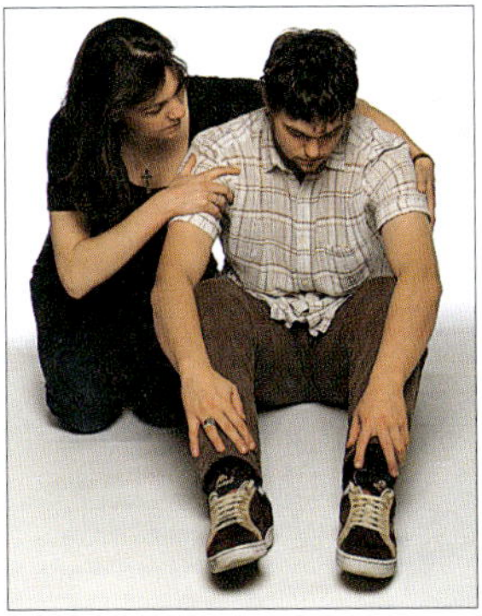

**If conscious**

1 Allow the casualty to assume the most comfortable position for himself.

NEVER give an unconscious casualty anything to eat or drink.

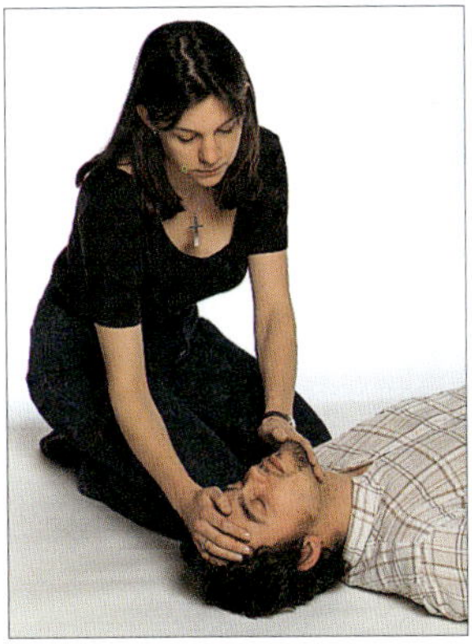

**If unconscious**

1 Check breathing and circulation regularly (*see page* 22). Be prepared to resuscitate with rescue breathing (*see page* 26) if breathing stops, and combine with chest compressions (CPR, *see page* 30) if there is no circulation.

2 If the casualty is breathing, place him in the recovery position (*see page* 34) and follow the ABC of resuscitation regularly (*see page* 21).

Even if adrenaline is administered, the casualty will still have to go to hospital, for observation and perhaps for further treatment. Adrenaline is used for an interim treatment; although it is very effective, it is not always enough to stop an anaphylactic reaction. Allergic reactions may cause the throat to close and you may have some difficulty establishing a clear airway. Continue resuscitation regardless, as some air may get through. Be prepared to give an injection of adrenaline to the casualty if he carries it and you know how to do it.

# AMPUTATION

An amputation occurs when a limb or part of a limb becomes severed from the body. The casualty will need urgent surgery to try to refix the limb to the body.

## WHAT TO DO

1 ☎ Call for an ambulance immediately, making it clear that there has been an amputation. Specialist staff will be ready to deal with the emergency.

2 Apply direct pressure to the injured part. Do not attempt to use a tourniquet or to stem the flow of blood in any other way.

3 Apply a dressing to the affected limb and be prepared to treat for shock (*see page* 46).

If a limb has been severed completely:

1. Wrap it carefully in a plastic bag or in cling film, taken from several lengths in to reduce the risk of infection.
2. Place it in a bed of gauze or cotton wool and then place the whole thing in a plastic bag or a bucket with crushed ice. Do not allow the limb to come in direct contact with the ice.

# ASTHMA ATTACK

Asthma has become so common in the Western world, and so easily treated, that its potential dangers have almost been forgotten. Asthma is a condition in which the muscles in the walls of the airway go into spasm, so that breathing is difficult or impossible. Most sufferers have the condition under control with inhalers or steroid tablets, but attacks can still occur. Most asthma attacks are caused by allergy, stress or infection; occasionally they occur for no obvious reason.

Some common symptoms include coughing, wheezing, breathlessness and a tight chest, all of which can cause extreme distress.

WHAT TO DO

1 ☎ If it is a first attack or the casualty is without medication, call for an ambulance.

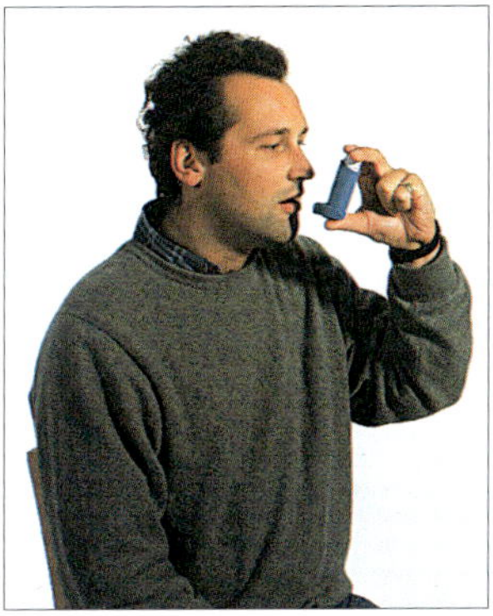

2 Allow the casualty to sit in an upright position. If he is more comfortable in another position, allow him to assume that position. Reassure him and keep him calm. Try to get him to breathe slowly and calmly.

3 If he has an inhaler or another form of medication, help him to use it.

☎ If the casualty does not respond immediately to the medication, and you have not already done so, call for an ambulance. Allow him to use reliever medication while you are waiting for the ambulance to arrive.

# BLEEDING AND WOUNDS

Wounds should only be addressed when you are certain that the casualty is breathing and has a circulation. If the wounds are serious, check circulation and breathing every few minutes while you are applying treatment (*see page* 22).

## *Small Cuts*

Any cut can provide a focus for infection, so it is important to clean the wound and apply a dressing as soon as possible.

WHAT TO DO

1 Make sure the casualty is seated and comfortable. Wash your hands.

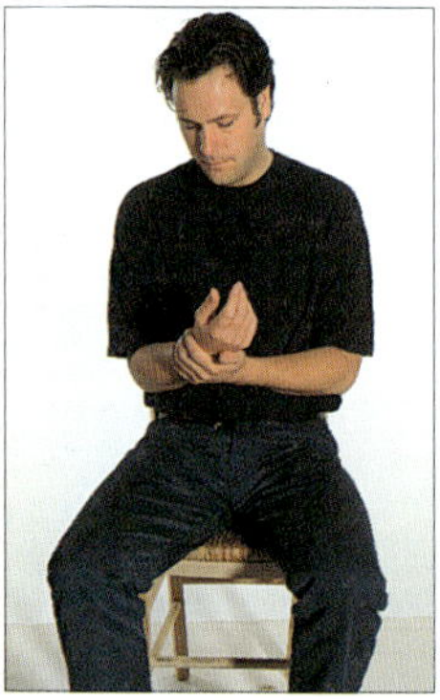

Because of the risk of HIV and other blood-transmitted diseases, wear disposable gloves wherever possible. Wash your hands in hot soapy water before and after contact with a bleeding casualty.

2 Gently clean the wound with gauze and cold running water. Clean around the wound with water and soap. Repeat this operation with gauze soaked in antiseptic.

It is important to clean away from the wound at all times, in short strokes. Use a fresh piece of gauze for each stroke. DO NOT continue washing the wound itself once a blood clot has started to form.

☎ DO NOT attempt to remove objects such as knives, sticks or glass (*see page 100*); call for an ambulance in this instance.

3 Remove any dirt from the wound.

4 Carefully dry the wound and dress it with an adhesive dressing (a plaster) or a sterile dressing (*see page 131*).

NEVER use cotton wool or anything fluffy or coarse to clean or dress a wound.

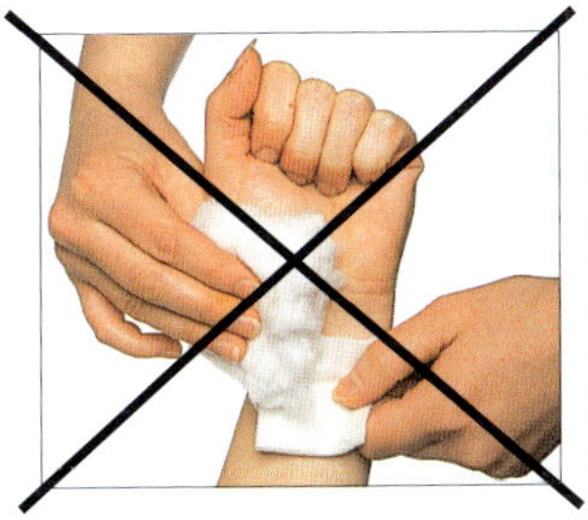

## *Gum and Socket Bleeding*

Bleeding which happens every time you brush your teeth is probably caused by gum disease, so arrange a dental check up to seek advice and treatment. Unusual bleeding soon after you've had a tooth out is probably from the socket and is more urgent.

WHAT TO DO

1 Roll up gauze or a small piece of clean fabric and place it over the entrance to the socket.

2 Press down on the pad to apply pressure to the socket and to stop the bleeding.

3 Do this for 10 minutes and then remove the pad carefully to see if the bleeding has stopped, taking care not to disturb the clot if you can. If it is still bleeding, repeat steps 1 and 2 and check again.

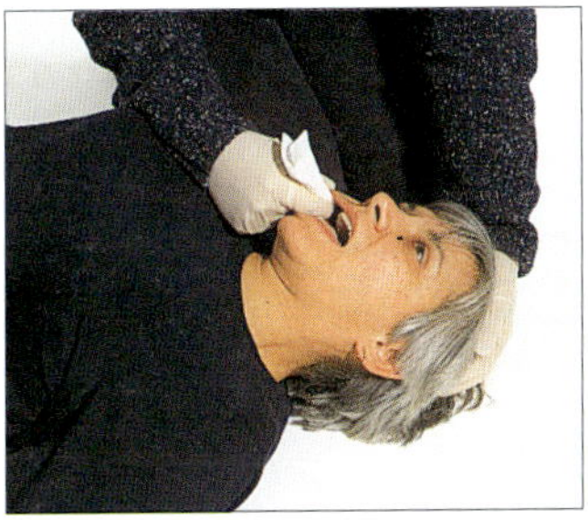

4 Bleeding usually stops after two or three attempts at this. If it doesn't, seek dental or medical advice immediately.

Any persistent bleeding that does not respond to First Aid treatment should be seen at a hospital or by a dentist.

## *Cuts to the Lips or Face*

There are arteries in the lips that can, if severed, cause profuse bleeding requiring emergency medical attention. Minor lacerations to the skin of the face (the cheeks, forehead, nose and chin, but not the eye area) can be treated in the same way.

WHAT TO DO

1 Place the edges of the wound firmly together with your finger and thumb, using a piece of gauze as a barrier between your fingers and the skin. This reduces the risk of infection.

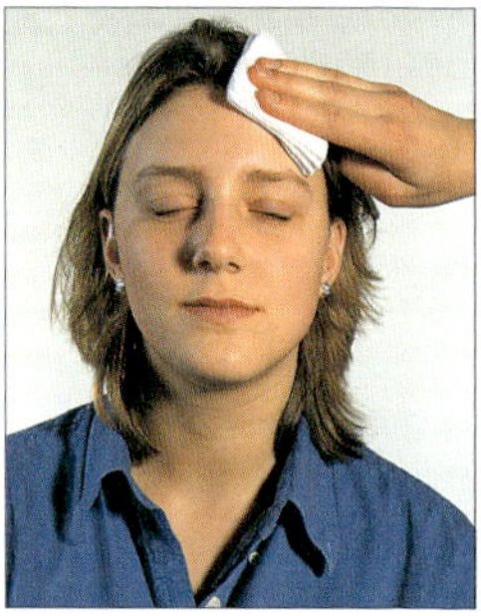

2 Apply pressure until the bleeding stops (probably about 10 minutes) or, if the wounds are severe, until medical help arrives.

## *Bruising*

A bruise indicates that there is bleeding under the skin or in the tissues, following an injury. A black eye is a bruise around the eye area and may be the result of a blow or injury to another part of the face or head. Always see your doctor if you have suffered a black eye.

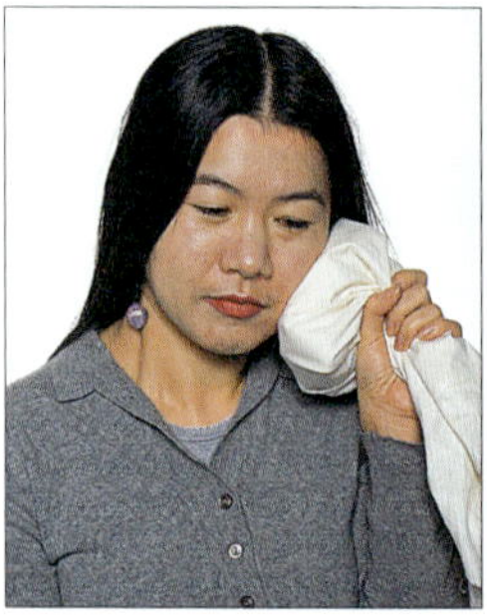

WHAT TO DO

1 A cold compress (*see page 134*), placed over the bruised area, will constrict the blood vessels and prevent further bleeding. It will also help reduce swelling and pain.

2 Ensure that the bruised limb or part of the body is supported, if that is possible.

## *Serious Internal Bleeding*

*(See page 45)*

## *Vaginal Bleeding*

*(See **Miscarriage**, page 101 and **Vaginal Bleeding**, page 102)*

## *Wounds to the Scalp*

*(See **Head and Neck Injuries**, page 94)*

## *Nosebleeds*

*(See page 122)*

## *Severe Bleeding*

*(See Haemorrhaging, page 93)*

# BURNS AND SCALDS

A burn is an injury to the skin and tissue caused by extreme heat or cold, by radiation (including sunlight), corrosive substances, electricity and friction. Scalds are burns which are the result of wet heat, such as hot water or vapours. See page 49 for the various types of burn.

The main priorities when treating burn victims are to:

- Ensure your own safety.
- Remove the casualty from risk of further burning.
- Provide resuscitation, if necessary.
- Provide rapid cooling.
- ☎ Call for an ambulance, explaining the type of burn (if known) and other information about the casualty that may help (extent of burns, position, age of casualty, etc.).
- Treat for shock or other injuries.
- Prevent risk of infection.

ABC of resuscitation (*see page 21*) is a priority. Get someone else to do the cooling while you begin the resuscitation.

For details on treating serious burns and scalds, and burns to the throat and mouth, *see pages 50–52*.

## *Miscellaneous Burns*

### MINOR BURNS

Minor burns are those that do not cover more than 9 per cent of the casualty's body, AND which are superficial.

WHAT TO DO

1 Protect yourself and the casualty from the source of the burn.

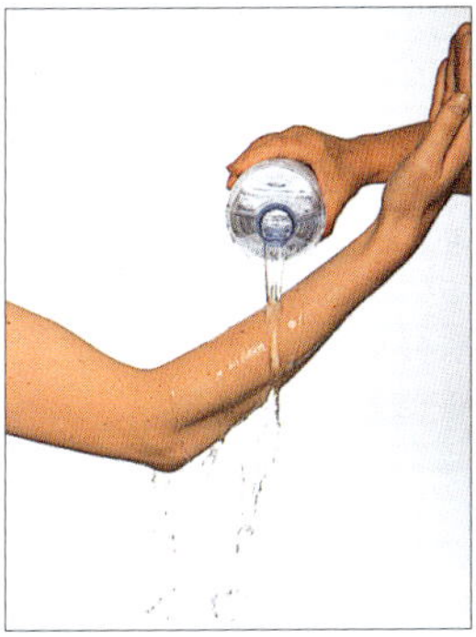

2 Cool the affected area with cold running water for at least 10 minutes.

3 Remove all constrictive clothing and jewellery if they inhibit the blood supply or if the possibility of swelling may make them difficult to remove later.

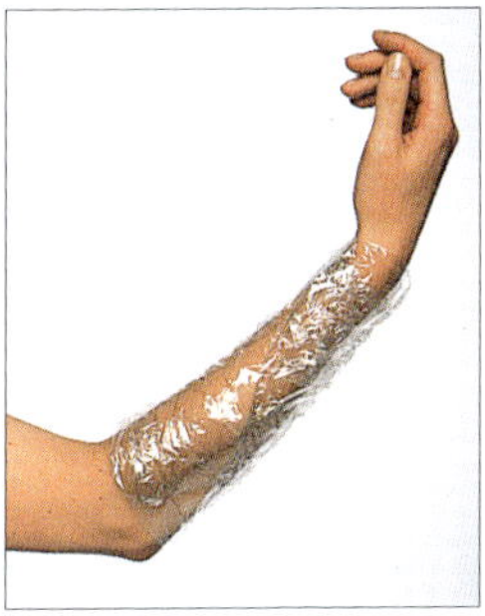

CLING FILM

4 Dress the burn with a sterile burns sheet, or any sterile (or very clean) fabric which is not fluffy. Loosely applied cling film, taken from several lengths into the roll, can be used.

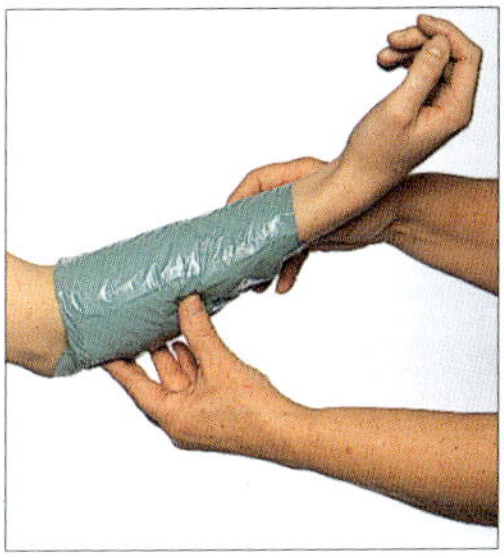

BURNS SHEET

NEVER wrap cling film tightly around a limb. The limb cannot swell and the circulation may become impaired.

NEVER use cling film unless the burn is cool – it will stick to the skin.

If you are concerned about the extent or severity of the burn, ensure that the casualty sees a doctor for treatment.

## *Chemical Burns*

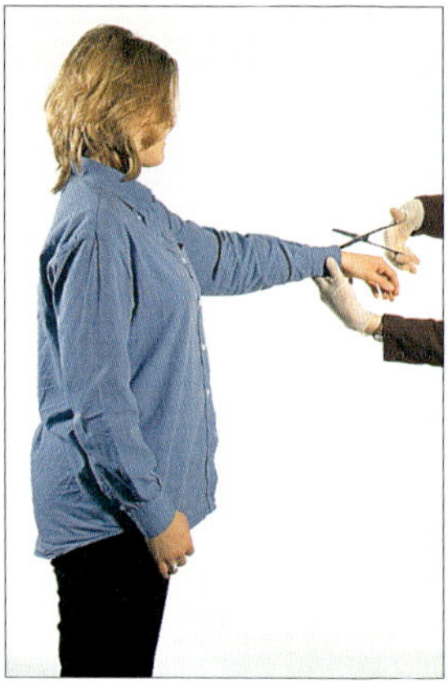

Chemical burns may result if the skin is exposed to household or workplace chemicals that are corrosive.

WHAT TO DO

1 Protect yourself from any dangerous chemicals.

**If conscious**

1 Remove or cut away clothing which may be saturated with chemicals (*see page 155*).

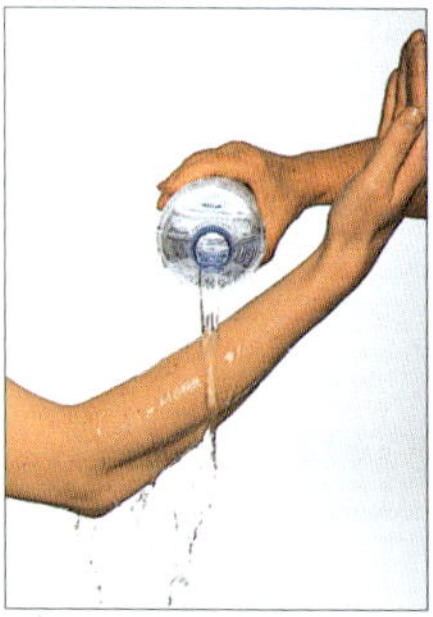

2 Cool the affected area with cold running water for at least 10 minutes.

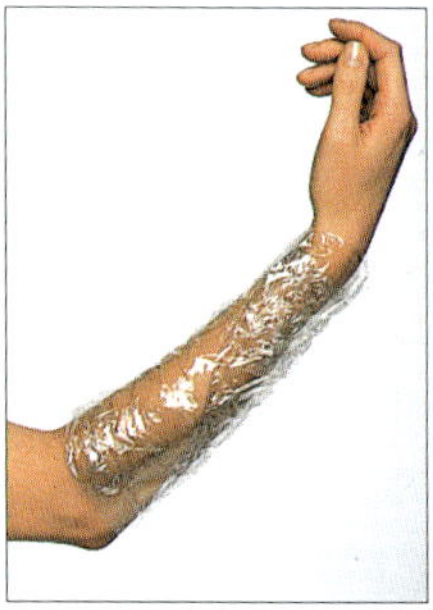

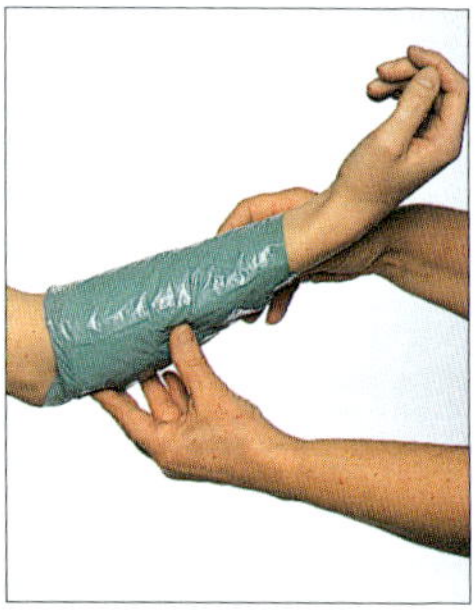

3 Protect the burn from infection with a sterile burns sheet, a clean bed sheet or pillowcase. In an emergency, cover the area with cling film, taken from several lengths into the roll to reduce the risk of infection.

4 Follow the ABC of resuscitation (*see page 21*), and check for signs of shock (*see page 46*).

**If unconscious**

1 Place the casualty in the recovery position (*see page 34*).

2 Follow the ABC of resuscitation (*see page 19*) before treating external burns (*see page 50*). Continue to check breathing and circulation, and watch for signs of shock (*see page 46*).

# *Electrical Burns*

Electrical burns are caused by an electrical current touching or running through the body. There may be no evidence of injury other than damage where the current entered and left the body, but internal damage may be extensive. Electrical burns may cause cardiac arrest (*see page 66*). The priorities are to:

- Switch off the electrical current, if possible.
- Follow the ABC of resuscitation (*see page 21*).
- ☎ Call for an ambulance or ask someone else to do this.
- Treat the burns and any shock (*see page 46*).
- Arrange for the casualty to be taken to hospital or make him comfortable until help arrives.

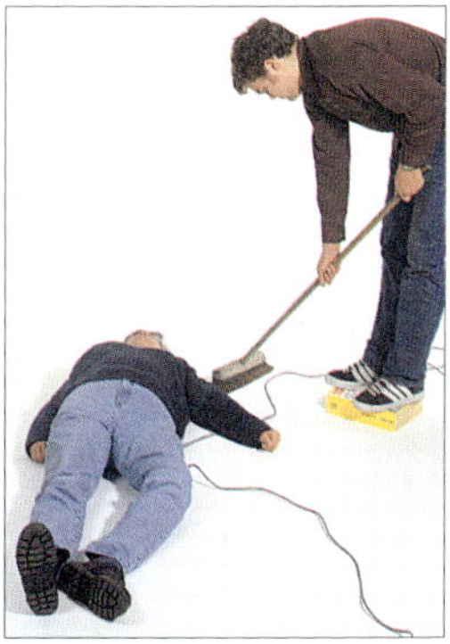

WHAT TO DO

1 Switch off the electrical current, if possible. Ensuring that you are in no danger yourself, remove the source from the casualty (*see page 80*).

**If conscious**

1 Treat the external burns (*see page 50*), and check breathing and circulation regularly.

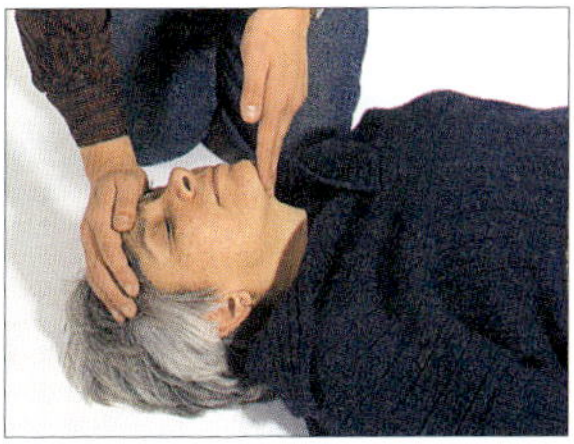

**If unconscious**

1 Follow the ABC of resuscitation (*see page 19*) before treating external burns (*see page 50*). Continue to check breathing and circulation, and watch for signs of shock (*see page 46*).

# CARDIAC ARREST AND HEART ATTACK

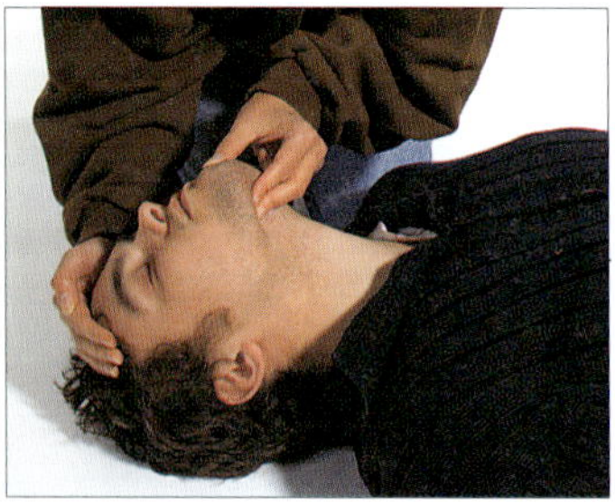

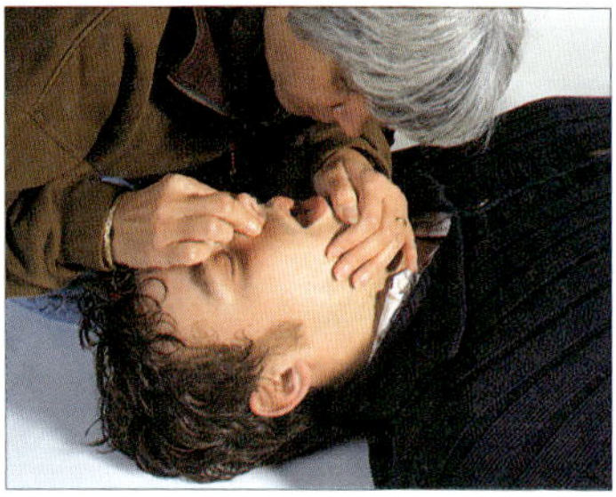

Heart attacks can cause 'cardiac arrest', when the heart actually stops beating. There will be no sign of a circulation and the patient will stop breathing. Other conditions, such as allergic reactions, blood loss, suffocation, electrical shocks and drug overdoses can also cause cardiac arrest.

A heart attack occurs when the blood supply to part of the heart itself is cut off in some way, usually the result of an obstruction, like a blood clot. This will cause severe chest pain and breathlessness when severe, but on occasions can produce no symptoms at all.

## Heart Attack

The symptoms of heart attack include:

- Breathlessness, faintness and anxiety.
- Pale, sweaty skin and blueness around the mouth and at the extremities.
- Weak, rapid pulse.
- Persistent crushing pain starting behind the breastbone and spreading around the chest like a tight band.
- Pain may radiate to neck, jaw and down arms (especially the left arm).
- Nausea and possible vomiting.

WHAT TO DO

**If conscious**

1 Seat the casualty comfortably, with legs and upper body supported.

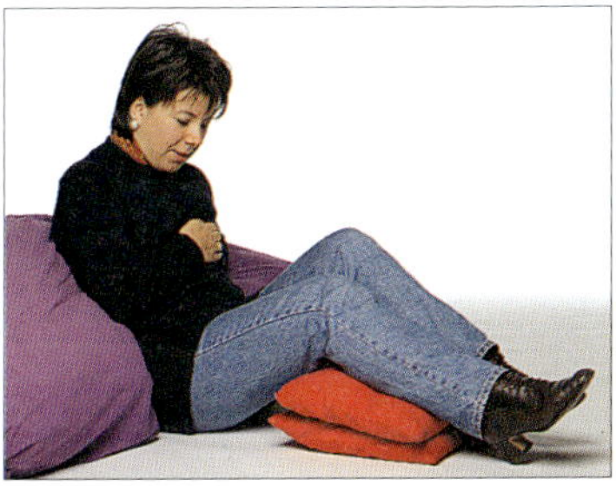

2 ☎ Call for an ambulance immediately.

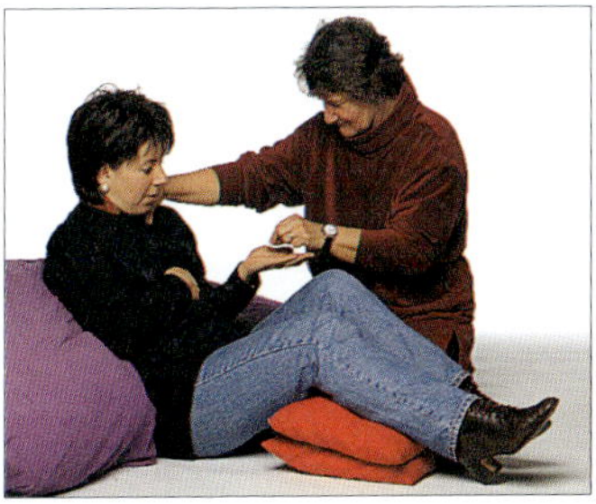

3 Offer the casualty one aspirin tablet to chew, but check that they are not allergic or on other medication which means they must not take aspirin.

4 Do not give them anything to eat or drink.

**If unconscious**

1 Follow the ABC of resuscitation (*see page 21*), and be prepared to resuscitate (*see page 26*).

# CHOKING

Choking occurs when a foreign body, such as a piece of food, becomes lodged in the airway, preventing air from reaching the lungs. Without an air supply, the body becomes starved of oxygen and brain damage and death will follow. A blocked airway is a serious medical emergency, and should be treated immediately.

Signs of choking include:

- The casualty clutching at her throat.
- Turning blue or very pale.
- Breathing with difficulty. Absence of breathing.
- Becoming unconscious within a few minutes.

> Most victims of choking cannot talk, but they will be able to respond if you give instructions. Ask a conscious adult if she is choking and try to persuade her to cough hard. Powerful inhalation will make the situation worse.

WHAT TO DO

**If conscious**

1 If coughing fails to dislodge whatever is blocking the airway, bend the casualty over.

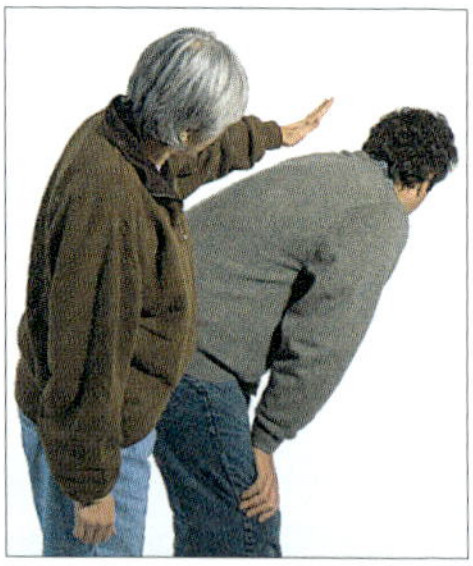

2 Give up to 5 hard blows on his back, between the shoulder blades, with the heel of your hand. If you do not get a response, move on to perform abdominal thrusts.

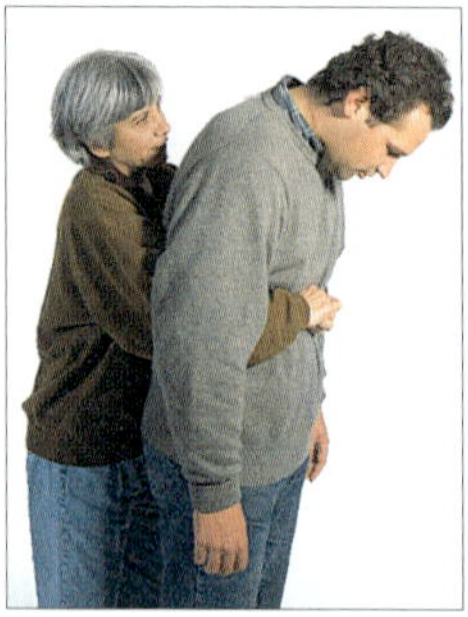

3 Try the abdominal thrust method (Heimlich Manoeuvre) (*see page 40*), up to 5 times. Alternate 5 back blows with 5 abdominal thrusts until the blockage is removed. This can be used on conscious or unconscious casualties.

BABIES

☎ A baby who is choking may turn blue and breathe noisily or not at all. You won't be able to ask her to confirm that she is choking, or to cough to eject the obstruction. Call for an ambulance immediately.

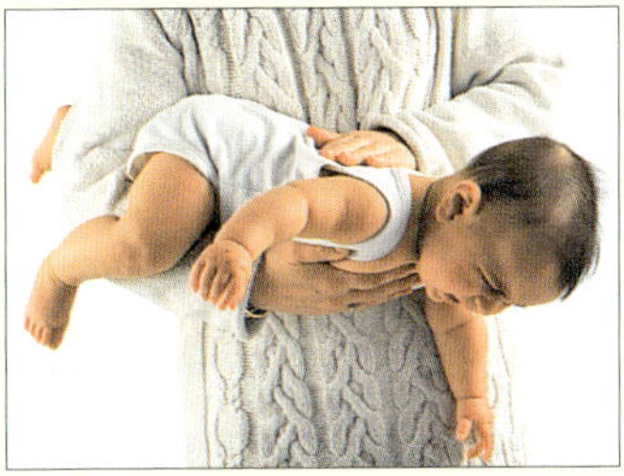

1. Lay the baby face down along your lower arm with his head supported in your hand.
2. With the heel of your other hand, deliver up to 5 back blows, just between the shoulder blades.

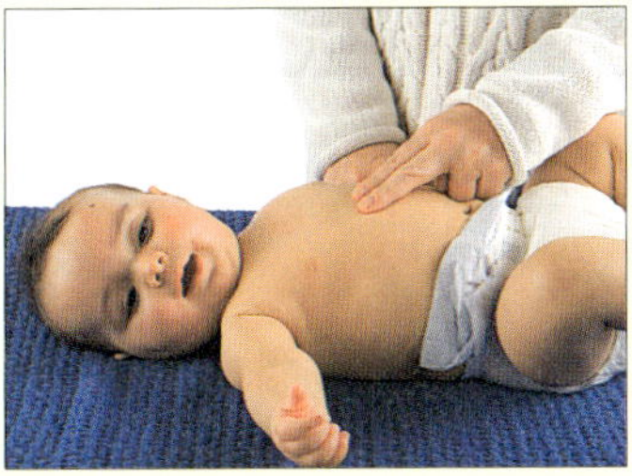

3. If he is still choking, turn him on his back along your other arm and support his head with your hand or place him on a flat surface.
4. Perform up to 5 chest thrusts (*see page 31*) and check in the mouth for visible obstructions.
5. Attempt up to 5 rescue breaths (*see page 28*).
6. Continue in cycles of 5 back blows, 5 chest thrusts, check mouth, 5 rescue breaths, until obstruction is removed or help arrives.

**Children**

A child who is choking may be able to confirm this, and she may be able to cough to eject the obstruction. If this does not work, follow these steps.

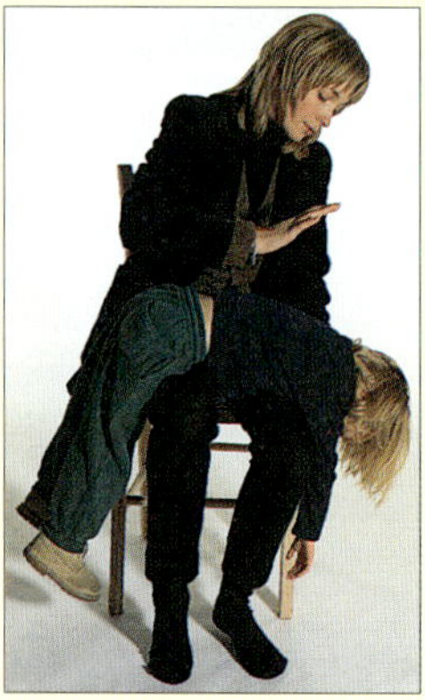

1. Lay a small child across your lap face down and deliver up to 5 back blows between the shoulder blades.
2. If the blows fail, perform up to 5 chest thrusts using a similar technique to chest compressions (*see page* 29) but a sharper, more vigorous action, and at a rate of about 20 per minute.
3. If these fail, give 5 more back blows followed by 5 abdominal thrusts, using just one hand.
4. Alternate back blows with abdominal or chest thrusts in subsequent cycles. Check to see if the airway is open with rescue breaths after each cycle.

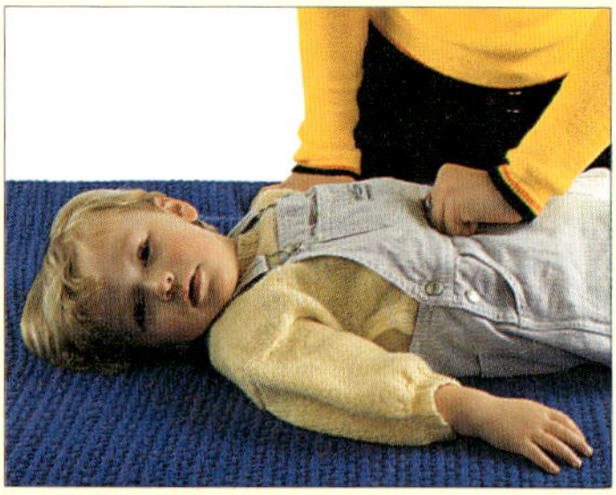

NEVER perform blind finger sweeps of the mouth as these may cause further damage. If the child does not breathe after 5 back blows and 5 chest thrusts, attempt to give 5 rescue breaths (*see page* 28). Check to see if the airway has cleared with rescue breaths after each cycle.

Act quickly. Starving the body of oxygen causes brain damage and eventually death. Call for help if you have any trouble clearing the throat, and continue treatment until it arrives.

# CONCUSSION

Concussion is caused by the brain being shaken inside the skull, usually as a result of a blow. Features of concussion include unconsciousness, vomiting, confusion upon wakening and occasionally temporary amnesia. Concussion can only be safely diagnosed when the casualty has wakened, for its main characteristic is that recovery will be complete.

WHAT TO DO

**If conscious**

1 Arrange for the casualty to see a doctor however well he feels. Beware of risk of neck injury.

**If unconscious**

1 ☎ Treat the casualty for unconsciousness (*see page 36*) and call for an ambulance.

2 Place the casualty in the recovery position (*see page 34*).

3 Check breathing and circulation regularly (*see page* 22)and take steps to treat wounds or fractures (*see pages 58, 81*).

# CONVULSIONS

Convulsions, also called fits, are contractions of muscles as a result of dysfunction of the brain. Convulsions are often a symptom of epilepsy, but there are a number of other causes, including:

- Injury to the head.
- Ingestion of some poisons, including alcohol in excess.
- Inadequate supply of oxygen to the brain.
- High temperatures (in children and babies).

There are many forms of convulsion, but the treatment is the same for all. Some convulsions are accompanied by unconsciousness (*see page 36 for treatment*).

> NEVER try to hold down someone suffering a convulsion.
> NEVER put your fingers or anything else into her mouth.

There are two common types of epilepsy – petit mal and grand mal.

## *Petit mal*

The episodes of this type of epilepsy may be so slight as to be unnoticed by an observer. The sufferer may appear to 'drift off', or to daydream. There may be twitching of the facial muscles, and other unusual responses, such as chewing with no food in the mouth, or making strange noises.

### WHAT TO DO

Treatment is aimed at making the sufferer comfortable and preventing her from causing damage to herself or others.

1 Sit her down quietly and provide reassurance.

2 Stay until symptoms have passed and she seems to be in control. Grand mal fits sometimes follow petit mal fits, so make sure she is not left alone.

## Grand mal

Grand mal epilepsy is more dramatic than petit mal, with often violent seizures and unconsciousness. There may be a warning to an attack, similar to that experienced with many types of migraine headache, called an 'aura', which is described as being an unusual sensation, smell or taste. In grand mal epilepsy, the attack is usually preceded by unconsciousness, and the sufferer may become blue in the face, with alarming convulsive movements of the muscles in the face and body. Breathing may stop altogether. The attack eventually ends and consciousness returns, although the sufferer may be confused and disorientated, and, perhaps, unaware of what has happened.

DO NOT force anything into the mouth to prevent them from biting their tongue.

DO NOT restrict, but guide their movements.

WHAT TO DO

Treatment is aimed at making the sufferer comfortable and preventing her from causing damage to herself or others.

1 Make sure that the sufferer is not injured while falling to the ground. Try to ensure she lies on her side to prevent problems if she vomits.

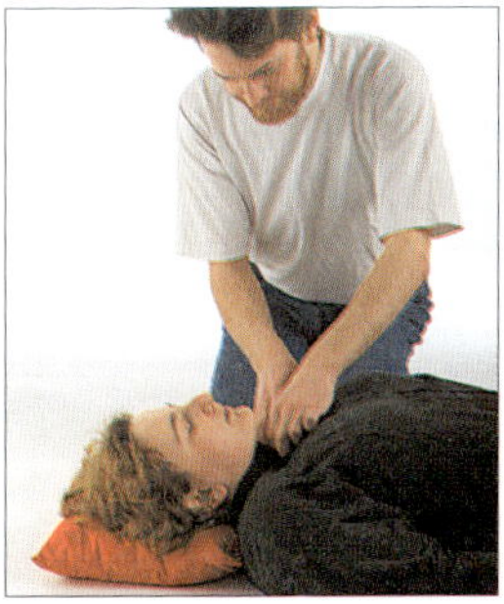

2 Loosen the clothing around her neck. Make sure there is nothing that will injure her within reach. Clear the area of onlookers.

☎ If the fit does not subside after 5 minutes, call for an ambulance.

3 When the convulsions stop, place her in the recovery position (*see page 34*). Do not leave her until she is feeling calm and well again. She may fall into a deep sleep. This is normal.

First-time sufferers should see a doctor. All sufferers should carry a Medic Alert bracelet or necklace.

# Febrile Convulsions

Febrile convulsions generally occur in children under five years old. They are the result of a high temperature, which interferes with the activity of the brain. All cases of high temperature and convulsions in small children should be taken to hospital; treated immediately, they should not cause any damage.

The priorities are:

- Protect the baby or child from anything which may cause injury; for instance, place her on the centre of the bed and watch her carefully.
- Keep her on her side to prevent problems if she vomits.
- Take steps to cool her in order to reduce the fever when the convulsion has stopped.
- ☎ Call for an ambulance.

> Don't be alarmed if breathing ceases for a few seconds and the baby becomes blue. This is normal. Unconsciousness should be treated immediately (*see page 36*). If breathing is not restored be prepared to perform CPR (*see page 31*).

## Cooling the child

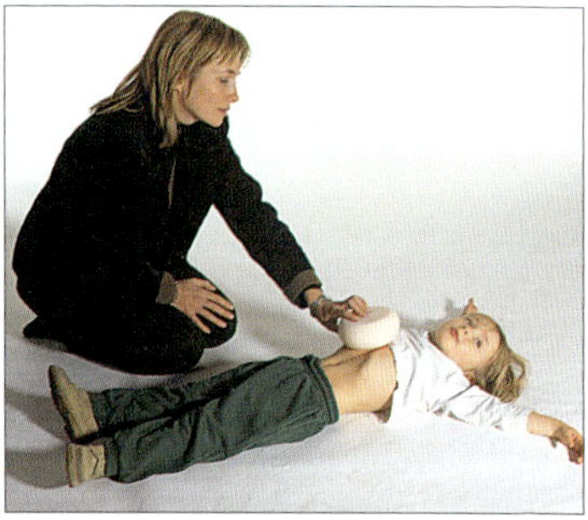

WHAT TO DO

1 Remove any constrictive clothing and place the baby or child in a safe place.

2 Sponge her all over with lukewarm water. Take care not to overcool.

3 ☎ Place her in the recovery position (*see page 34*), if possible, and call for an ambulance.

> If the baby or child becomes unconscious, prepare to resuscitate (*see page 28*).

# CRUSH INJURIES

Crush injuries are normally the result of a heavy weight falling onto the casualty, although they can also occur in car accidents and other high-velocity accidents, such as train or aircraft accidents.

☎ Call for an ambulance immediately. Serious kidney damage can result from the effects of crush injuries, and expert medical assistance at an early stage is of vital importance.

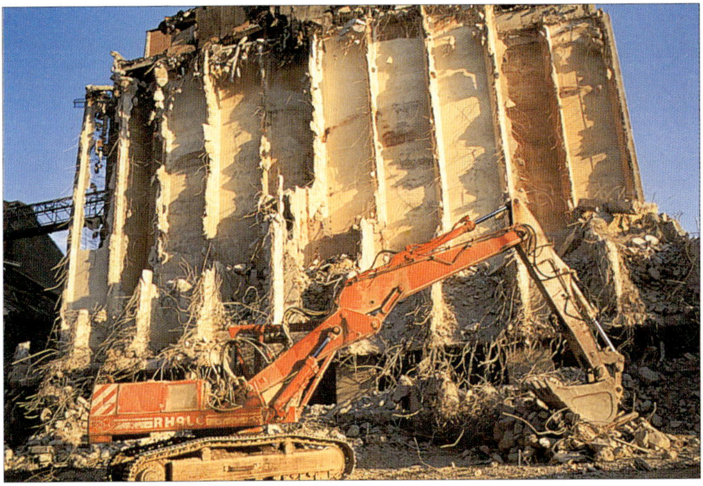

Crush injuries can be sustained when a substantial weight falls onto a person, such as scaffolding or rubble on a building site.

Characteristics of a crush injury include:

- An obvious weight across a portion of the body.
- Bruising, pain and swelling at the site of the injury.
- Reduced or non-existent pulse below the site of injury.
- Cold and pale limbs below the site of injury.
- Shock (*see page 46*).
- Possible fractures.

WHAT TO DO
Treatment depends on how long it has been since the injury was sustained.

## Less than Ten Minutes After the Accident

DO NOT attempt to remove the weight if you might drop it back onto the casualty.

DO NOT move the casualty unless vital.

If the casualty becomes unconscious, treat (*see page 36*) and place in the recovery position (*see page 34*) until help arrives.

1 ☎ Call for an ambulance.

2 Remove the weight as quickly as possible.

3 Follow the ABC of resuscitation (*see page 21*) and then assess injuries.

4 Take steps to control bleeding (*see page 43*) and treat for shock (*see page 46*).

5 Tell the emergency medical team when it arrives how long the casualty was crushed for.

## Ten Minutes or More After the Accident

DO NOT remove the weight unless it is lying on the chest.

1 ☎ Call for an ambulance.

2 Reassure the casualty, staying with him until help arrives, and follow steps 3–5 above, if required.

# DIABETES

There are two problems which may occur in diabetics:

- **Hypoglycaemia**, which is a severe drop in the blood sugar level;
- **Hyperglycaemia**, which occurs when the blood sugar level is too high.

*See page 36* for signs that a casualty is diabetic.

## *Hypoglycaemia*

Hypoglycaemia can be caused by an overdose of insulin, anti-diabetic tablets, too much exercise or insufficient carbohydrate intake and can develop very quickly. It is characterised by:

- Feelings of faintness, with shaking and occasionally shivering.
- Confusion and occasionally aggression.
- Appearance of being drunk.
- Dizziness, sweating and pale skin.
- Possible loss of consciousness leading to coma.

WHAT TO DO

**If conscious**

1 Give refined carbohydrates immediately, in the form of food or drink. Chocolate, fizzy drinks and sweets are good choices.

2 ☎ If there is no improvement after 15 minutes, call for an ambulance.

**If unconscious**

1 ☎ Place the casualty in the recovery position (*see page 34*). Call for an ambulance immediately.

## *Hyperglycaemia*

Hyperglycaemia is normally caused by inadequate insulin intake. It is characterised by:

- Sweet smell of casualty's breath.
- Feeling unwell for some time.
- Possible loss of consciousness.

WHAT TO DO

1 ☎ Call for an ambulance, and if the casualty becomes unconscious, follow the ABC of resuscitation (*see page 21*).

# DROWNING

Death by drowning can occur in just inches of water. Casualties who have been presumed drowned, their bodies starved of oxygen for up to 30 minutes, have recovered with no ill-effects whatsoever. As long as it does not present any safety risk to you, attempt to save and resuscitate anyone who is drowning or presumed drowned.

WHAT TO DO

1 Without risking your own safety, remove the casualty from the water, if possible performing mouth-to-nose rescue breathing as you bring her to dry land (*see page 26*). Bring her closer to land or to the side of the pool, between breaths.

2 On dry land, remove her from the water as quickly as possible and cover with one blanket.

3 Follow the ABC of resuscitation (*see page 21*).

4 Ensure help is on its way.

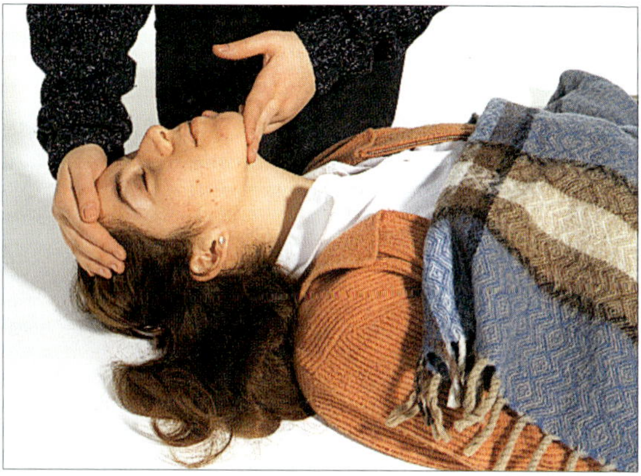

**If conscious**

1 Place the casualty in the recovery position (*see page 34*). Ensure that she is warm. Check for signs of hypothermia (*see page 90*) and treat accordingly.

2 Stay with her, checking breathing and circulation regularly until help arrives.

**If unconscious**

1 Clear the airway (*see page 24*) and check for breathing. If there is no breathing, give 2 rescue breaths (*see page 26*).

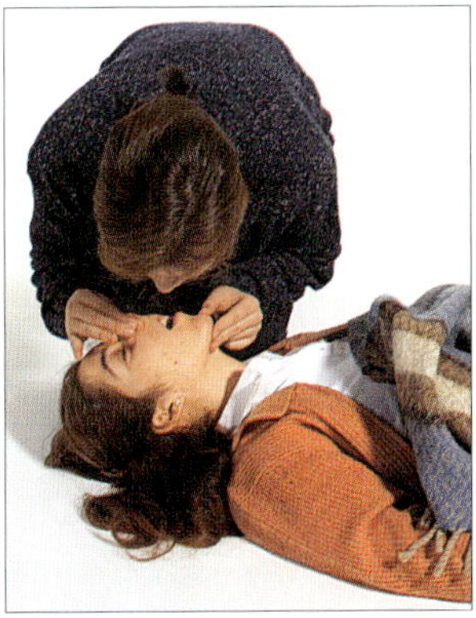

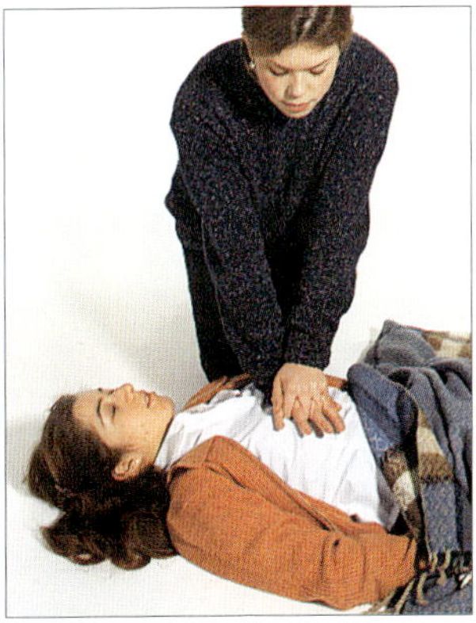

2 ☎ Check the circulation and if there is none, begin CPR (*see page 30*). If you are sure there is a circulation, perform rescue breathing only, and recheck circulation every minute. If you are alone, call an ambulance after about one minute. If you are with someone, send them straight away.

3 If the casualty starts to vomit, turn them on their side to allow it to drain freely.

Be prepared to continue CPR for as long as it takes to get the casualty to hospital.

# ELECTRIC SHOCK

There are two types of electrical shock – high-voltage and low-voltage current. High-voltage current shocks are often fatal, and if they are not, it is usual for the casualty to have been thrown some distance by the contact and therefore to have sustained other injuries and burns. Low-voltage current shocks are usually caused by an electrical appliance or power point.

Only use water to cool burns when you are certain that the electrical supply has been disconnected.

## *High-voltage Injuries*

☎ All power must be cut off before you make any attempt to approach the casualty. Even then great caution must be employed. High-voltage electricity could leap as far as 18 metres (60 feet), so it is best to call for the emergency services immediately, and keep the area clear.

## *Low-voltage Injuries*

WHAT TO DO

1 Before doing anything, make certain that the current has been disconnected at the mains. If you are unable to reach the mains, disconnect at source (the electrical socket).

2 In the event that there is still a current present, you should take care to stand on something that will not conduct – paper or anything wooden or rubber.

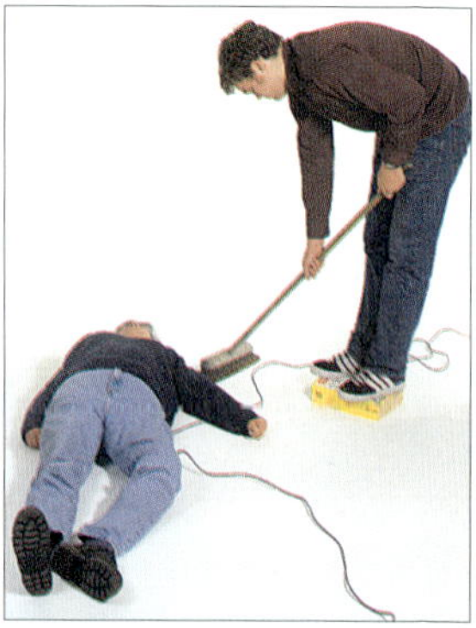

3 Push the source away from the casualty with a broom handle or a chair. Use something made of non-conducting material.

4 Follow the ABC of resuscitation (*see page 21*) and be prepared to resuscitate if necessary (*see page 26*).

5 ☎ Call for an ambulance.

6 Treat burns (*see page 49*). Check the ABC of resuscitation.

# FRACTURES

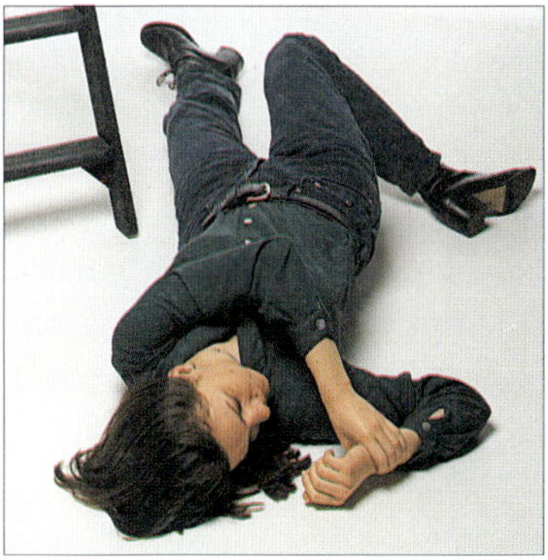

There are two types of fracture:

- **Closed**, where the skin is unbroken and the bone is not susceptible to infection.
- **Open**, where the bone is visible or protrudes from the skin through a wound, making it susceptible to infection.

Fractures occur as a result of force or stress on the bone itself. Older people, particularly women, and anyone suffering from conditions like osteoporosis, where there is a loss of bone density, are more susceptible to fractures.

Unless the bone is obviously protruding from the flesh, you may not be aware of a fracture. Signs include:

- Pain, swelling and occasionally bruising at the site of the fracture.
- Inability or reluctance to move the affected part.
- Grating sensation or sound when movement is attempted.

## *Closed Fractures*

DO NOT attempt to move the casualty if a closed fracture is suspected, until you have secured and supported the affected limb or part.

WHAT TO DO

1 Support the affected part above and below the injury so that the fracture itself cannot move. If possible, fasten the injured part of the body to another, uninjured part with a bandage or sling (*see pages 135–46*).

2 ☎ Call for an ambulance.

3 Treat for shock (*see page 46*).

# Open Fractures

☎ You can identify an open fracture because there is a wound at the site. There will be two courses of action, depending on whether or not the bone is protruding. Always call for an ambulance before performing any First Aid.

## Protruding Bones

WHAT TO DO

1 Cover the wound with a sterile cloth or piece of gauze. If you have nothing sterilised, then anything clean, such as a handkerchief, will do.

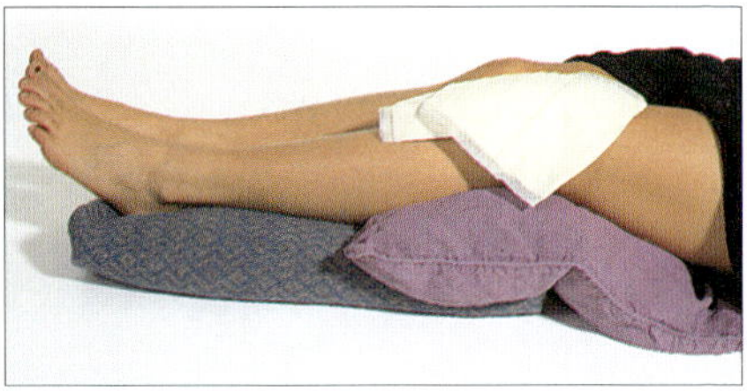

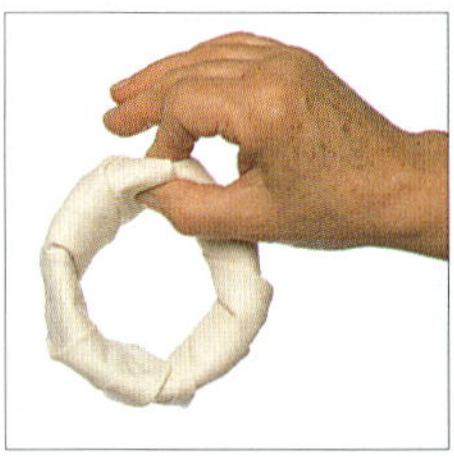

2 Line the wound with a ring of cloth or gauze (roll it to get this effect) and place this over the gauze or cloth.

3 Fix this in place with a larger bandage, placed diagonally across the fracture site.

4 Immobilise the injured part by tying or fastening it to an uninjured part of the body (*see page* 86).

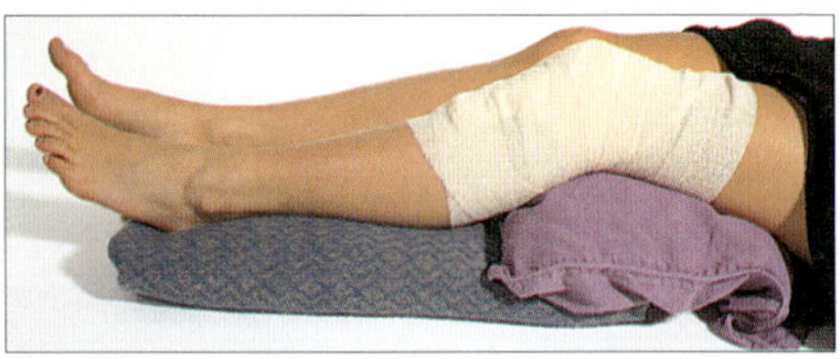

5 Wait for the ambulance.

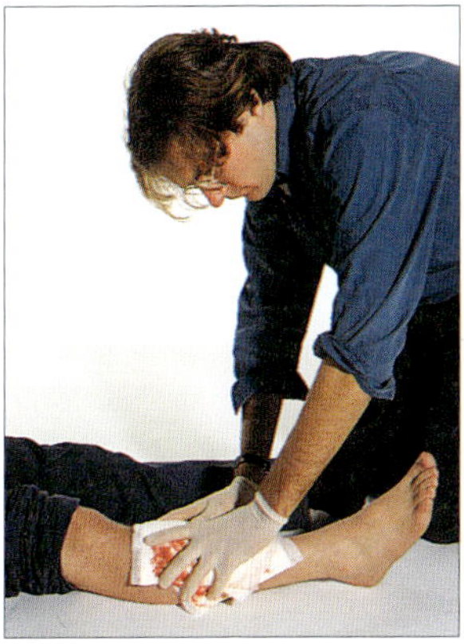

## No Protruding Bones

WHAT TO DO

1 If there is bleeding, firmly but carefully apply pressure to the sides of the wound, squeezing them together so that bleeding will be controlled.

2 With a piece of sterile gauze, or, failing that, a clean cloth, cover the area and secure with a firm bandage (*see page 135*).

3 Immobilise the injured part by tying or fastening to an uninjured part of the body, if possible.

4 Wait for the ambulance.

# *Facial Fractures*

Fractures of the nose, cheekbone and jaw may be distressing and cause bleeding from the mouth, nose and ears. There may be severe swelling, pain on opening the jaw and trouble speaking or swallowing.

WHAT TO DO

1 Make sure the airway is clear and that the casualty is able to breathe (*see page 24*).

2 Place the casualty in a forward position so that any blood, vomit or saliva will run out.

3 ☎ Call for an ambulance.

4 Treat any bleeding (*see page 43*).

FOR A BROKEN NOSE:

- Gently apply a cold compress (*see page 134*) to the injury.

FOR A BROKEN JAW:

- Hold a pad against the jaw and support it with your hand until help arrives.

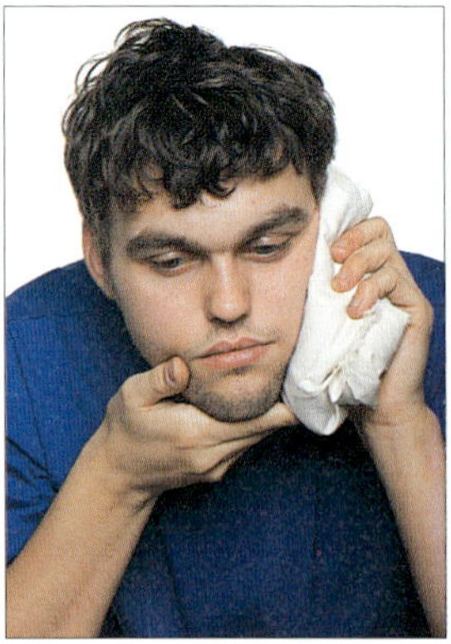

## *Fractured Kneecap*

Signs will include severe swelling and pain in the knee area, and tenderness over the kneecap itself.

WHAT TO DO

1 Place the casualty so that the head and shoulders are supported, but she is comfortably reclined.

2 If possible, straighten the affected leg gently.

Straightening the affected leg will be very painful. Do not try to force the knee into a completely straight position.

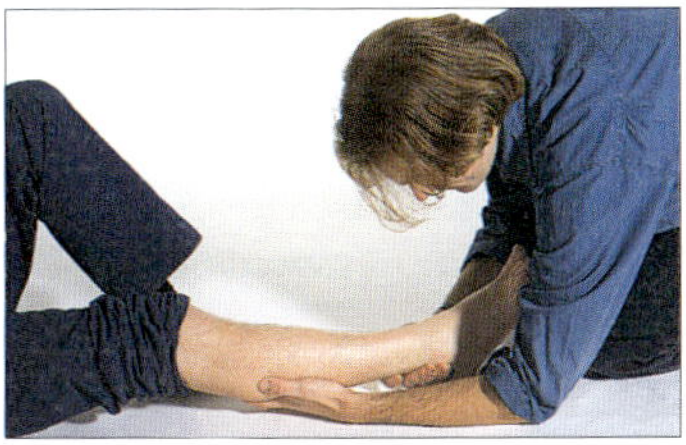

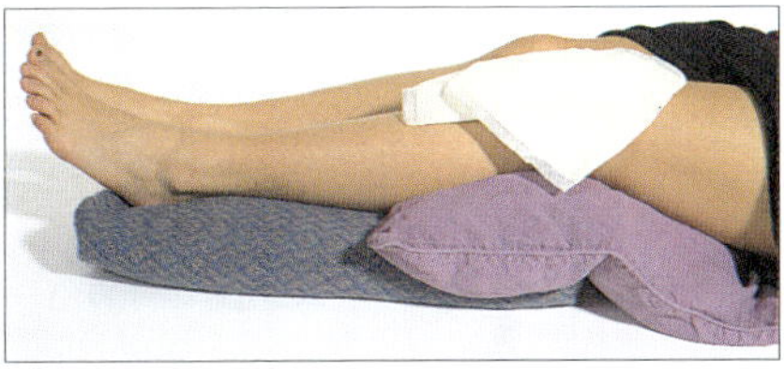

3 Elevate the leg and slip a padded board or anything firm, like a large book, under the knee and place extra padding under the knee itself.

4 Wrap more padding around the joint and bandage it into place (*see page 139*).

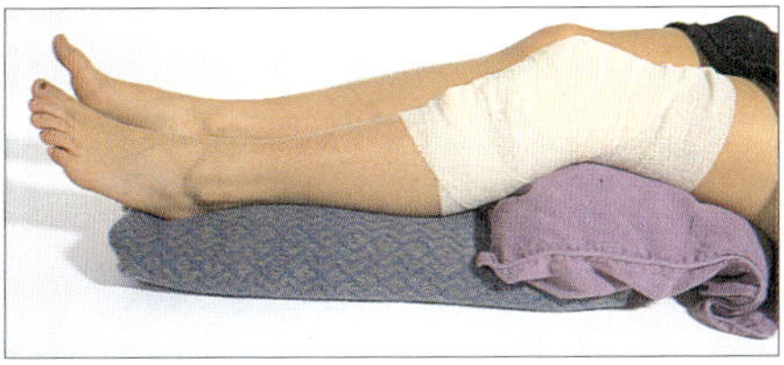

5 ☎ Call for an ambulance.

# Fractured Leg

A fractured leg may show signs of severe bruising. This sort of injury often leads to shock in the casualty. There may be signs of deformity and swelling.

DO NOT move the legs unless absolutely necessary, and remember that there will be severe pain and a risk of shock (*see page 46*).

WHAT TO DO

1 ☎ Call for an ambulance. If the casualty is unconscious, follow the ABC of resuscitation (*see page 21*) and be prepared to resuscitate, if necessary.

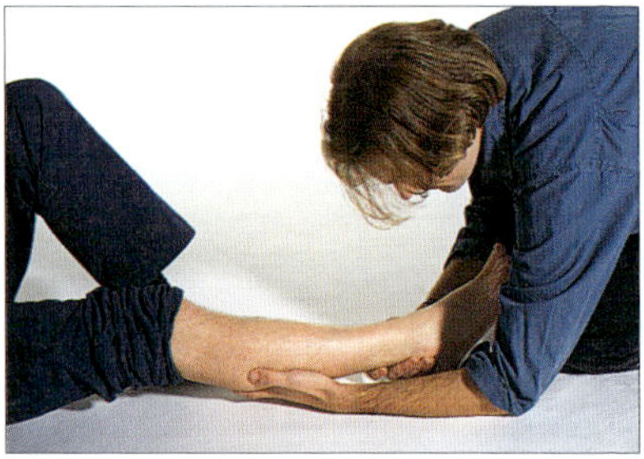

2 Very gently straighten the leg, if possible.

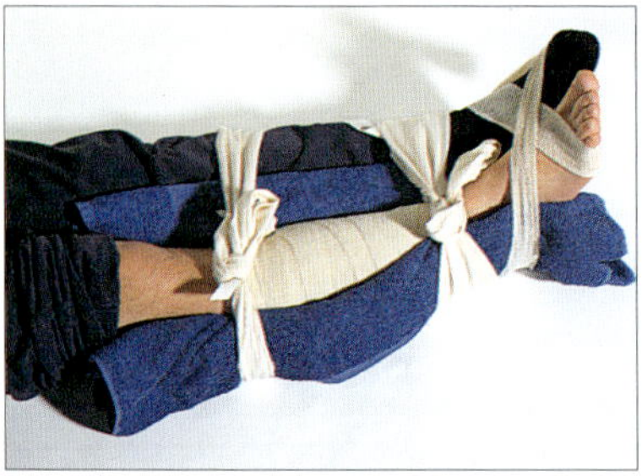

3 Carefully treat any bleeding (*see page 43*).

4 Immobilise the leg by placing a rolled-up towel or the equivalent on either side of the leg and then bandage both legs together. Make sure the knots of the bandage appear on the uninjured side.

5 Hold the feet together with a bandage tied firmly at the foot.

6 Wait for the ambulance.

## Fractured Collarbone

There are two collarbones, which sit at the top of the ribcage, between the breastbone and the shoulders. A fractured collarbone will be painful, particularly on moving the arm on that side.

WHAT TO DO

1 Seat the casualty comfortable in an upright position, and place the arm on the injured side across the chest, supporting the elbow with another hand.

2 Support the arm with an elevation sling (*see page 146*) and secure the arm to the chest with a broad bandage (*see page 140*).

3 Arrange for transportation to hospital.

## Fractured Arm

Fractures of the arms are common and vary in severity. The arm may be broken at the upper part, the elbow, or the lower arm. Fractured arms are characterised by an inability to perform normal movements, pain that increases upon movement, and occasionally, deformity.

WHAT TO DO

1 Seat the casualty comfortably in an upright position.

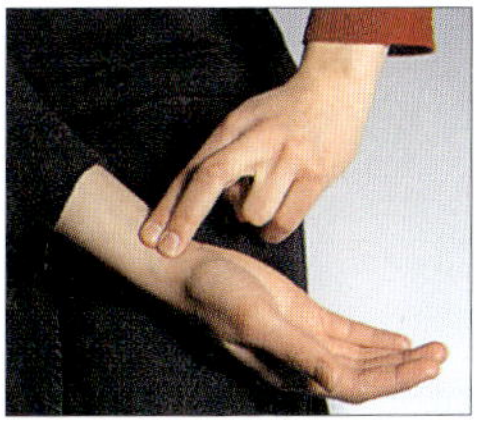

2 ☎ Check for a wrist pulse, and if there is none present, call for an ambulance.

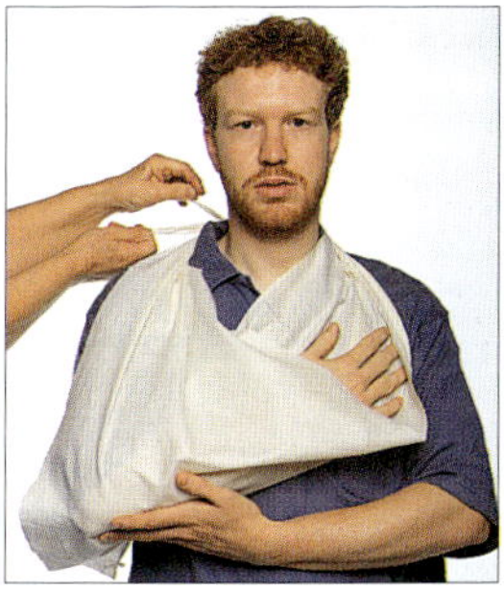

3 Very gently lay the forearm of the injured arm across the casualty's chest and ensure that it is well supported while you place padding between the chest and the arm, and on both sides of the injured arm. A rolled-up towel or coat can be placed on the casualty's lap for extra protection and support.

4 Carefully place the arm in a sling (*see page 145*), and secure the arm to the chest with a broad bandage (*see page 140*).

5 Wait for the ambulance, if you have called for one, or arrange for transportation to hospital.

## *Fractured Hand or Fingers*

There are a number of small bones in the fingers, wrist and hand, and fractures to these bones are very common. Symptoms include bleeding, bruising or swelling. Movement will be painful and difficult. Most casualties will be unable to form a fist.

WHAT TO DO

1 Remove any rings, if possible, before swelling becomes a problem.

2 ☎ Deal with any bleeding (*see page 43*), and ensure that there is a circulation in the wrist (*see page 22*). If none is present, call for an ambulance.

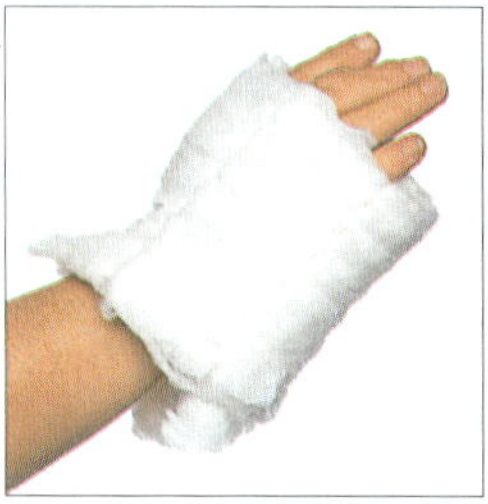

3 Apply padding around the hand and wrist, taking care not to move them unnecessarily.

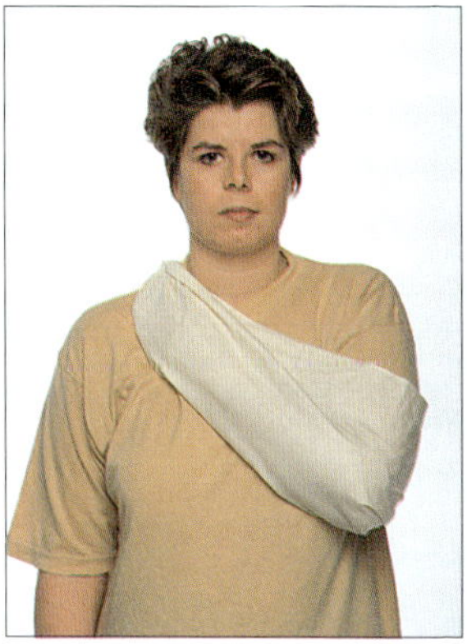

4 Carefully place the arm in an elevation sling (*see page 146*), and raise it so that the hand is above the level of the elbow. Fix the sling with a broad bandage (*see page 140*).

5 Wait for the ambulance or arrange for transportation to hospital.

## *Fractured Ribs*

Features of one or more fractured ribs include:

- Sharp pain on breathing in; trouble with breathing.
- One side of the chest may move in when the victim inhales and move out when he exhales. This is called paradoxical breathing and causes serious respiratory problems.
- Occasionally blood from the mouth, either coughed up or vomited.
- Blueness around the mouth.

WHAT TO DO

1 Strap the arm on the injured side to his chest and arrange for transportation to hospital immediately.

Fractured ribs may be accompanied by a penetrating chest wound, also called a 'sucking wound'. A wound of this nature prevents the lung on the injured side from properly inflating, because air is drawn into the wound when the victim breathes in. This is a serious condition and steps to seal the wound must be taken immediately. Place an airtight dressing over the wound and secure it on 3 sides only.

## *Fractures of the Head, Neck and Back*

☎ NEVER move a casualty with suspected head, neck or back injuries, for fear of causing further injury and possibly paralysis. You must always call for an ambulance first, and then reassure the casualty until help arrives.

If the casualty is unconscious, follow the ABC of resuscitation (*see page 21*), taking care to move the casualty as little as possible. The airway should be cleared, if possible, by lifting the chin only without tilting the head. Avoid moving the head from side to side.

# FROSTBITE AND HYPOTHERMIA

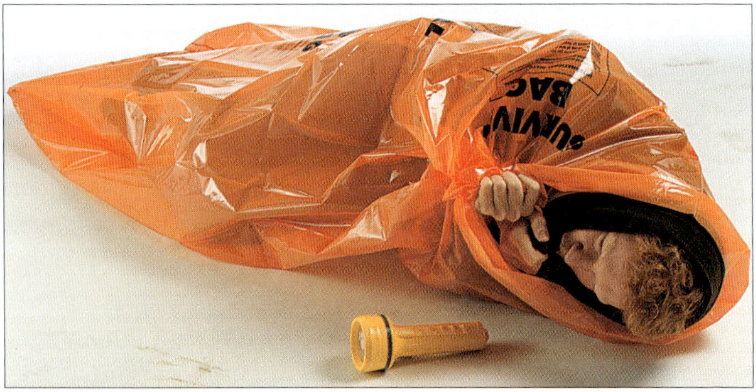

## *Frostbite*

Frostbite occurs when the tissues in parts of the body become frozen, preventing blood flow to the area. The extremities are most susceptible to freezing, in particular, the fingers and toes, and the tips of the ears and nose. Frost-bitten skin becomes white and hard, then swollen and red. In extreme cases it can result in gangrene.

### SUPERFICIAL FROSTBITE

Symptoms include:

- Slight pain/ burning sensation
- Numbness
- Skin grey/yellow

### DEEP FROSTBITE

Symptoms include:

- No feeling
- Waxy appearance
- Hard to touch

### WHAT TO DO

Both types of frostbite should be treated in the same way.

1 Move the casualty to a warm place, or one that is sheltered from the elements.

2 Warm the affected area to body temperature (37°C or 98.4°F) e.g. in your armpit or crotch. Do not massage the area or attempt to move it.

3 As soon as possible, seek medical attention. Look for signs of hypothermia (*see opposite*) and prepare to treat.

# Hypothermia

Hypothermia occurs when the body temperature falls below normal (37°C or 98.4°F). It is most common in the elderly and people who are thin or hungry, and it occurs when the body is unable to maintain heat. Hypothermia can be caused by long-term exposure to cold (in an unheated house, for instance), or by short-term contact while swimming, for instance, or spending time out-of-doors.

Symptoms include:

- Intense shivering that ceases as the casualty becomes colder.
- Slow pulse and rate of breathing.
- Drowsiness that will eventually fall into unconsciousness and perhaps to a coma.
- Low body temperature that continues to drop.
- Cold, dry skin, occasionally blueness around the mouth.
- Eventually, heart failure.

## WHAT TO DO

☎ The first priority in all cases of hypothermia is to call for an ambulance.

### INDOORS

**If conscious**

1 Place the casualty in a warmed bed. Climb in with her to provide your own body warmth, if possible. Cover her head with blankets so heat does not escape.

2 Provide warm drinks and food.

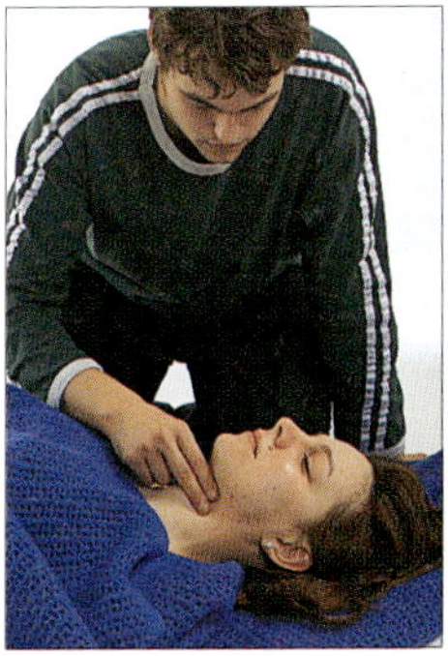

3 Check breathing and circulation regularly (*see page* 22).

**If unconscious**

1 Follow the ABC of resuscitation (*see page* 21) and prepare to resuscitate (*see page* 26).

NEVER give an unconscious casualty anything to eat or drink.

- NEVER massage a victim of hypothermia or allow any unnecessary movement.
- DO NOT use hot-water bottles or hot baths to warm the casualty.
- NEVER use more than one blanket and your own body heat to warm the casualty.
- NEVER give brandy or other alcohol in an attempt to warm the victim.

OUT-OF-DOORS

**If conscious**

1 Ensure that the casualty is taken to a sheltered area or indoors as soon as possible.

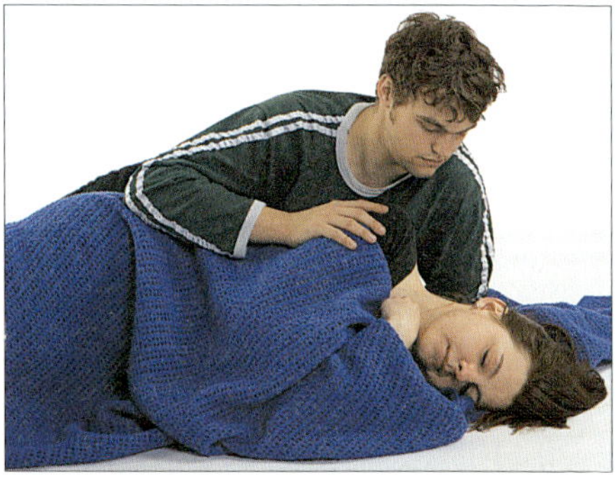

2 Using one blanket for cover and your own body for warmth, lay the victim down and then lie next to her yourself.

3 Offer warm food and drinks, if available.

**If unconscious**

1 Follow the ABC of resuscitation (*see page 21*) and be prepared to resuscitate (*see page 26*).

It is important to note that a casualty of hypothermia may appear dead when actually in a deep coma. Brain damage is often prevented by cold temperatures, because the metabolic rate of the body becomes slower, so oxygen deprivation may have had a less serious effect. Always attempt resuscitation.

# HAEMORRHAGING

Haemorrhaging is any bleeding from or in the body. Severe blood loss is a serious condition and must be considered a medical emergency. External bleeding should be controlled as much as possible (*see page 44*) and the casualty taken to hospital. Internal bleeding is more difficult to pinpoint, but suspected cases also need urgent medical attention (*see page 45*).

There are some general points to remember about bleeding:

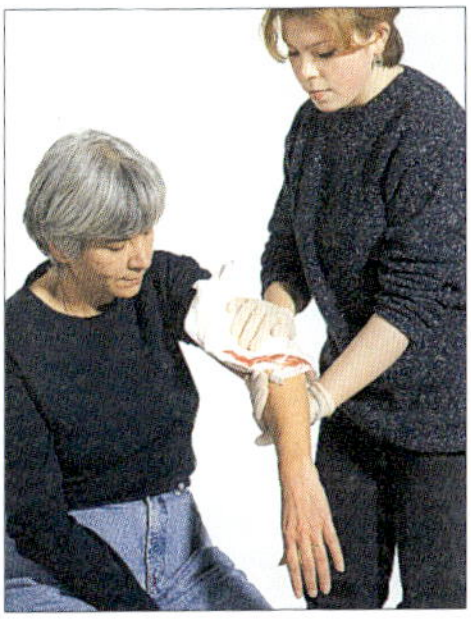

1 Unless there is something embedded in a wound you should apply direct pressure, ideally with a clean pad under your hand.

2 The injured part should be raised so that it is above the level of the heart. Lay the casualty down, if at all possible.

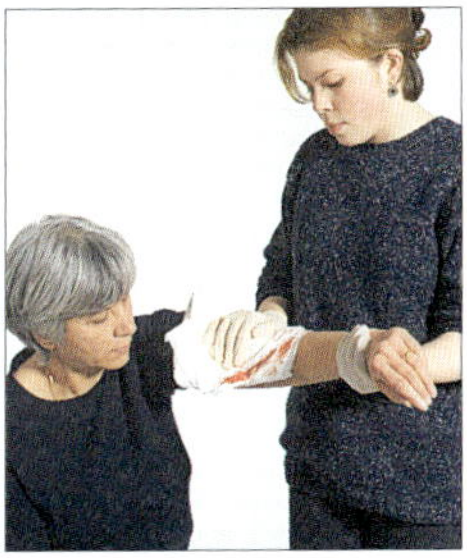

Dressings should always be sterile or as clean as possible to reduce the risk of infection.

3 ☎ Call for an ambulance.

4 Check for signs of shock (*see page 46*) and treat accordingly.

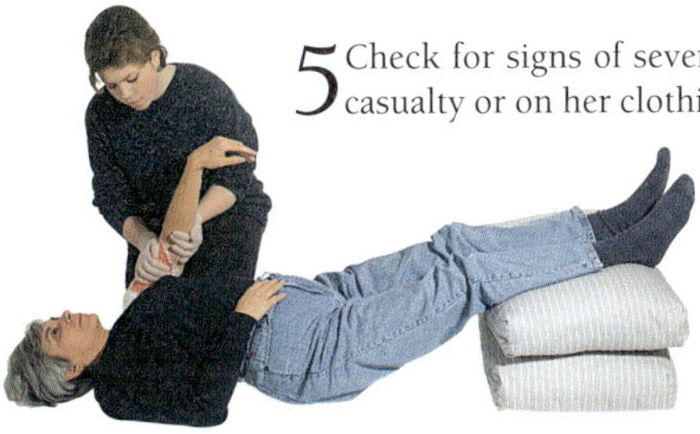

5 Check for signs of severe blood loss (around the casualty or on her clothing, *see page 43*).

6 If internal bleeding is suspected, raise the casualty's legs and keep her warm until help arrives.

7 Follow the ABC of resuscitation (*see page 21*) and be prepared to resuscitate (*see page 26*).

# HEAD AND NECK INJURIES

Head and neck injuries can be serious and require medical attention. Any blow that causes bruising or bleeding may also have caused concussion and fracture (see below). There may be no external signs of injury at all and in an unconscious victim it is often difficult to assess the extent and nature of the injuries.

DO NOT move the casualty if you suspect a spine or neck injury.

## *Concussion*

*(See page 71)*

## *Fractured Skull*

Signs of a suspected skull fracture include facial discoloration, bleeding from the nose or ears, bleeding from the scalp and abnormal dilation of the pupils.

☎ If there is an open fracture of the skull (*see page 89*), there is a serious risk of infection and complications. Call for an ambulance.

WHAT TO DO

**If conscious**

1 Lay the casualty down in a comfortable position, with the head and shoulders slightly elevated.

2 ☎ Call for an ambulance.

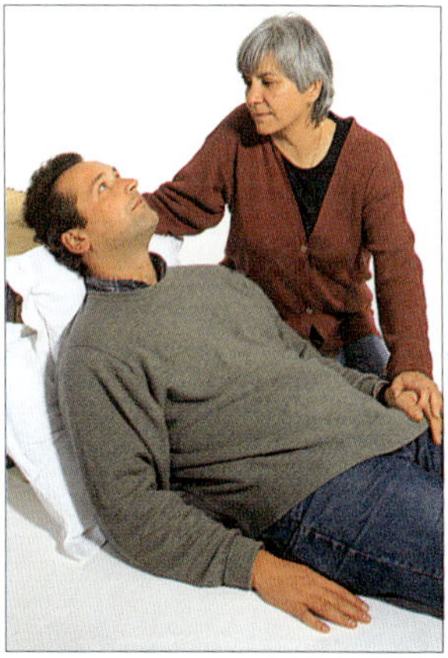

3 Treat any wounds (*see page 58*). If there is bleeding from the ear, do not attempt to place any pads in the ear canal, but wrap a pad against the outside of the affected ear and position the casualty so that the ear is turned downwards.

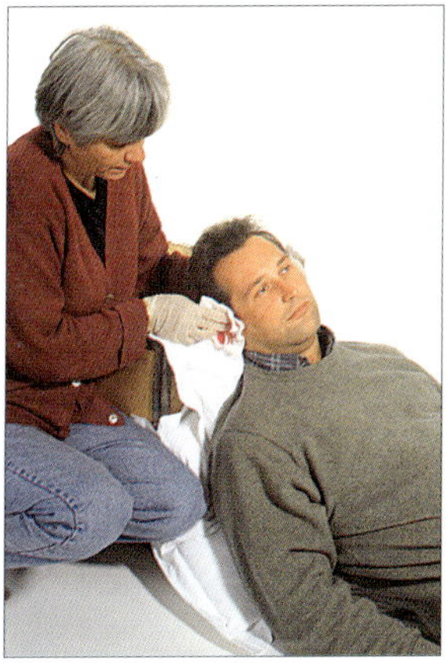

4 Check the casualty for signs of shock and treat accordingly (*see page 46*).

5 Provide reassurance until help arrives. Check breathing, circulation and responses (*see page 22*) regularly and be prepared to resuscitate (*see page 26*).

**If unconscious**

1 Follow the ABC of resuscitation (*see page 21*) and be prepared to resuscitate (*see page 26*).

2 ☎ Call for an ambulance.

3 If the casualty starts to vomit, place him in the recovery position (*see page 34*) and check breathing, circulation and responses (*see page 22*) every few minutes.

# Scalp Wound

Your first priority is to prevent the loss of blood and to prevent bacteria from gaining access to the wound. Remember that a scalp wound may be indicative of something much more serious, such as a skull fracture, so do not press too hard when stopping the bleeding. Watch carefully for signs of further injury.

WHAT TO DO

1 Wash your hands carefully and place a clean (sterile if possible) pad over the wound itself, ensuring that firm, direct pressure is used at all times.

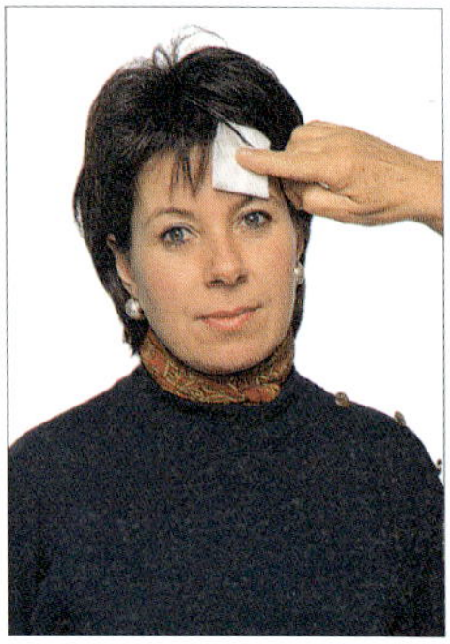

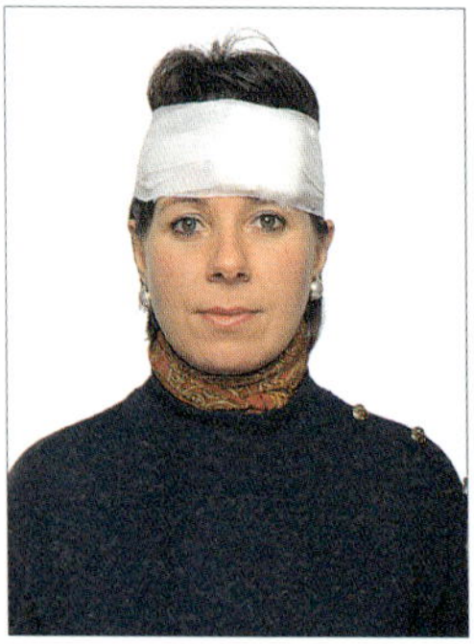

2 Secure the pad with a triangular bandage (*see page 140*).

**If conscious**

1 Lay the casualty down in a comfortable position with the upper body slightly elevated.

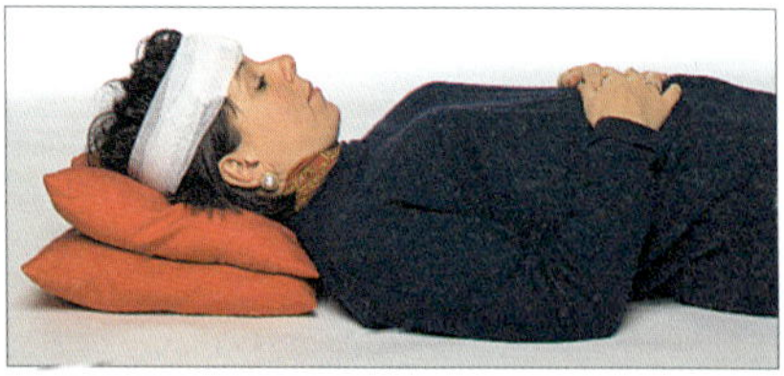

2 Check breathing, circulation and responses (*see page 22*) every few minutes until help arrives. Be prepared to resuscitate (*see page 26*).

**If unconscious**

1 Follow the ABC of resuscitation (*see page 21*) and be prepared to resuscitate (*see page 26*).

2 ☎ Call for an ambulance.

# Fractured Neck

A fractured neck may be characterised by stiffness and an inability to move the arms or legs. There may be pain and tingling at the site of the fracture. There may be no clinical indication at all. Suspicion is vital.

DO NOT move the casualty unless her safety is jeopardised.

DO NOT remove a crash helmet (*see page 158*) unless the airway or breathing is obstructed or if it is necessary to resuscitate (*see page 21*).

**WHAT TO DO**

1 ☎ Call for an ambulance.

**If conscious**

1 Hold the casualty's head still until help arrives.

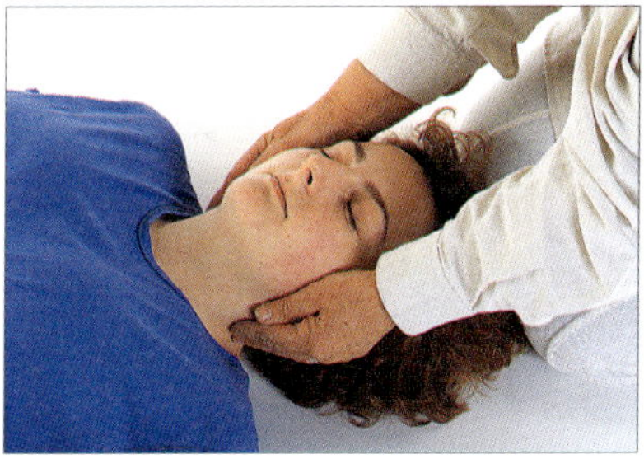

**If unconscious**

1 Follow the ABC of resuscitation (*see page 21*) taking care not to move the neck. Be prepared to resuscitate (*see page 26*). Continue to check breathing, circulation and responses (*see page 22*) regularly.

# HEAT EXHAUSTION AND HEAT STROKE

When exposed to extreme heat, the body is unable to maintain its normal temperature and loses its ability to function properly. The two conditions that develop from this are heat exhaustion and heat stroke.

## *Heat Exhaustion*

The process leading to heat exhaustion is more subtle than heat stroke. It may occur following exercise, or it may happen in climates where the air is hot and humid which means that sweat is unable to evaporate and cool the body. Heat exhaustion is the result of loss of body fluids, and is common among travellers exposed to unaccustomed heat, especially if they are also suffering from diarrhoea and vomiting. Symptoms include:

- Dizziness and confusion.
- Nausea.
- Profuse sweating.
- Leg cramps.
- Weak pulse and shallow breathing.
- Fatigue.

WHAT TO DO

**If conscious**

1 ☎ Call for an ambulance.

2 Lay the casualty down out of direct sunlight, preferably in the shade or in an air-conditioned area. Raise the legs above the level of the heart, using a pile of books or clothing.

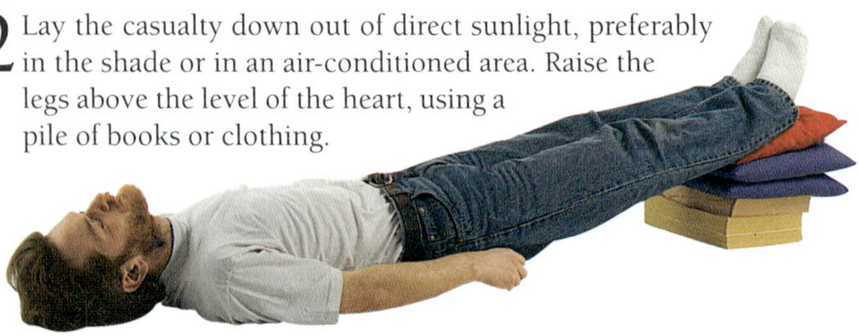

3 Give a cool non-alcoholic drink to sip. Your First Aid kit may have an electrolyte substance that will help replace lost body salts. Alternatively, something like Lucozade or Gatorade is appropriate. If that is not available, try adding 1 teaspoon of salt and 4 teaspoons of sugar to one litre (2 pints) of cool water or orange juice.

**If unconscious**

1 Follow the ABC of resuscitation (*see page 21*) and be prepared to resuscitate (*see page 26*). Place in the recovery position (*see page 34*) if the casualty is breathing.

2 Check breathing and circulation (*see page 22*) regularly.

## *Heat Stroke*

Heat stroke is more serious than heat exhaustion and comes on much more suddenly. It can be caused by exposure to high temperatures, particularly those in a humid environment, but it can also result from a high fever (*see page 127*). In heat stroke, the part of the brain which controls temperature fails to work and dysfunction in many parts of the body occur. Symptoms include:

- Severe headache and dizziness – this is occasionally mistaken for migraine in sufferers.
- Hot reddened skin.
- High temperature (above 40°C or 102°F).
- Nausea.
- Rapid strong pulse.
- Confusion, leading to unconsciousness.

WHAT TO DO

**If conscious**

1 ☎ Call for an ambulance.

2 Move the casualty to a cool place – preferably sheltered or air-conditioned.

3 Dampen a sheet with cold water and wrap it round the casualty. Continue to wet the sheet until her temperature drops. Do not remove the sheet until the temperature is normal.

4 When the temperature has dropped, cover her with one sheet and monitor breathing and circulation until help arrives.

**If unconscious**

1 Follow the ABC of resuscitation (*see page 21*) and be prepared to resuscitate (*see page 26*). Place in the recovery position (*see page 34*) if the casualty is breathing.

# IMPALEMENT

An impalement occurs when a foreign object sticks into the body. Under no circumstances should you try to remove the impaling object.

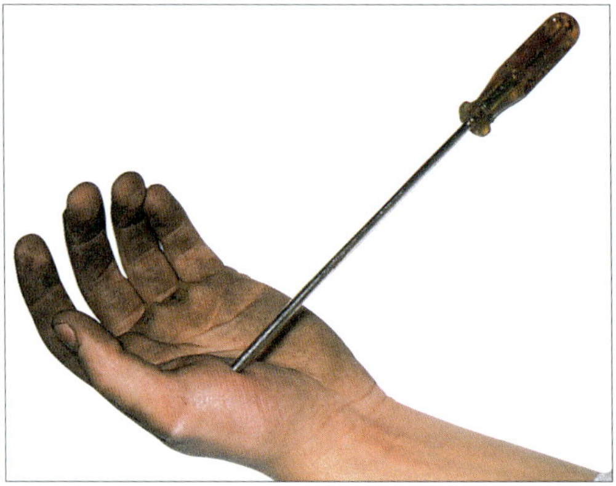

WHAT TO DO

1 ☎ Call for an ambulance immediately, providing as many details as possible about the nature of the injury.

2 Reassure the casualty and if possible, try to support his weight so that he is more comfortable.

3 Support the impaling object so that it is not moved.

# MISCARRIAGE

A miscarriage is the loss of a baby before the twenty-fourth week of pregnancy. A threatened miscarriage occurs when a pregnant woman experiences any of the symptoms of miscarriage but does not expel the foetus. A woman who is miscarrying is likely to have vaginal bleeding and possibly abdominal cramps. Heavy bleeding may lead to shock (*see page 46*). The casualty is likely to be very distressed.

> In any case of miscarriage – threatened or complete – you must seek medical advice.

WHAT TO DO

1 Lay the casualty down with her head and shoulders slightly raised. Make sure she is comfortable and reassure her. She may be embarrassed about her condition, so be discreet.

2 Offer a clean towel to deal with the blood and let her fix it herself.

3 Check for signs of shock (*see page* 46), and check her breathing and circulation (*see page* 22) regularly.

4 ☎ If the bleeding is profuse, call for an ambulance. If she is bleeding only slightly, call a doctor.

5 Stay with the casualty until help arrives and provide as much reassurance as she will allow.

> In a miscarriage the foetus and the placenta will be expelled. If this occurs while you are with the casualty, place it out of her sight but safe for later examination. Do not be surprised if she wants to see the foetus – many women do.

If the casualty has acute abdominal cramps, is dizzy and faint, has pain in her shoulders and there is a chance that she is pregnant, whether she is bleeding or not, this could mean an ectopic pregnancy. An ectopic pregnancy is when a foetus develops outside the womb, usually in a Fallopian tube; it is often misdiagnosed as appendicitis or irritable bowel syndrome and it is a serious life-threatening condition that must be treated at once. Arrange for transportation to hospital immediately.

## *Vaginal Bleeding*

Bleeding from the vagina which is not related to the menstrual cycle may indicate a number of conditions, some of which will not respond to any first aid measures. Miscarriage may be a possibility in some cases (*see page 101*). Always remember that the casualty is likely to be very embarrassed about the situation and you should remain calm and courteous throughout the procedure.

WHAT TO DO

1 Clear the area or remove the casualty to a more private place.

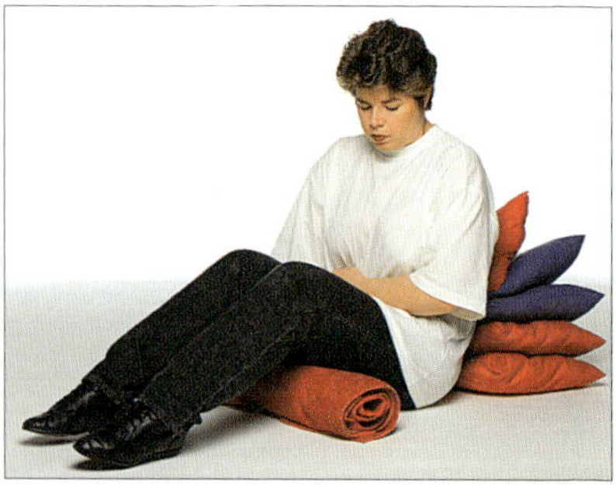

2 Offer a clean towel or sanitary pad to help staunch the flow of blood.

3 Lay her in a comfortable upright position with her knees bent.

4 ☎ If the bleeding is severe and undiagnosed, call for an ambulance.

Severe bleeding may lead to shock (*see page 46*). Be prepared to treat.

# POISONING

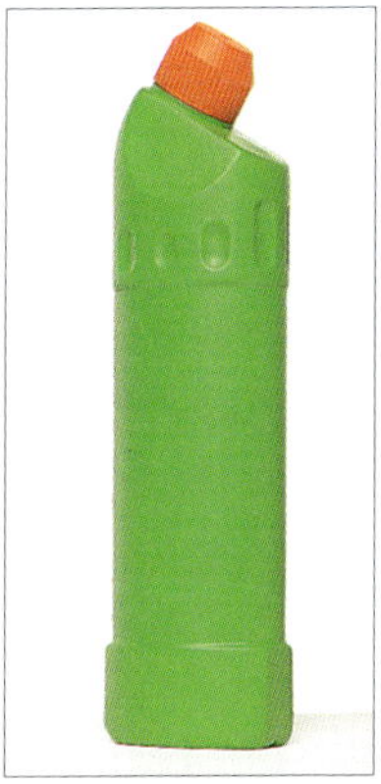

Household bleach

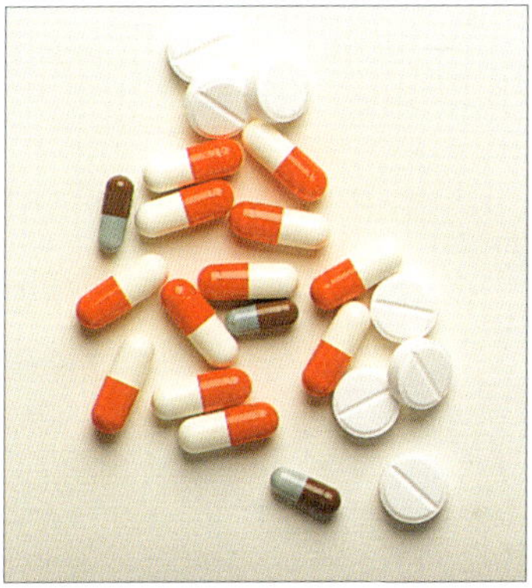

Tablets

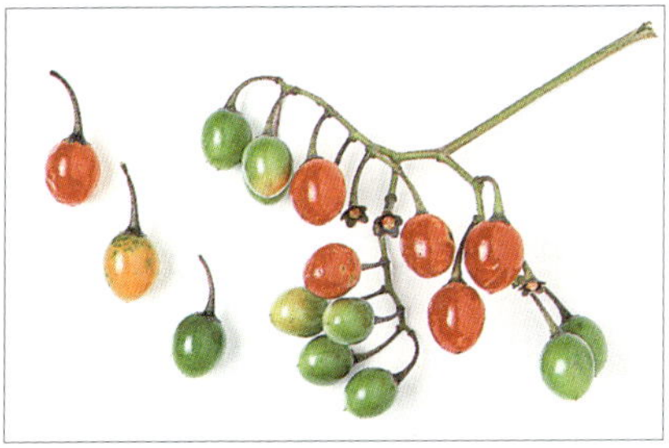

Woody nightshade (*Solanum dulcamara*)

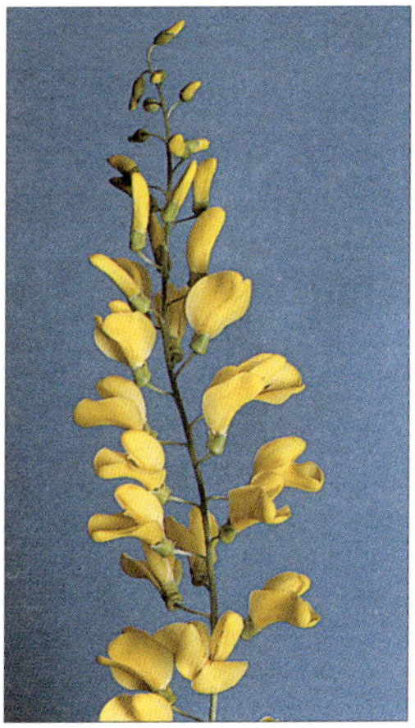

Laburnum

Poisoning is one of the most common emergency situations, and one for which the majority of people are ill-prepared. It is usually accidental, but it can occasionally be deliberate, as in a suicide attempt. Most accidental poisoning occurs from taking an overdose of drugs or alcohol, or by eating tainted food. Many people – children in particular – are poisoned by household cleaners, by medication, by garden plants and chemicals used in the garden, and by fluids such as antifreeze and methylated spirits and by gases and rodent poisons.

There are some key points to remember in any case of poisoning:

- Do not waste time trying to find an antidote.
- ☎ Call for an ambulance or advise the hospital that you are bringing in the casualty.
- Provide as much information about the poison as you can, so that they are prepared for your arrival.
- Do not try to make the casualty vomit.
- If the casualty shows signs of having taken a corrosive poison and he is conscious, get him to drink milk or water so that if he does vomit the poison will be less concentrated.

WHAT TO DO

1 Get help immediately.

> Ensure that any traces of poison are washed from the mouth and face before performing rescue breathing. Consider performing mouth-to-nose breathing (*see page 27*) if the casualty's mouth is contaminated.

2 Follow the ABC of resuscitation (*see page 21*) and be prepared to resuscitate (*see page 26*) .

3 Both conscious and unconscious breathing casualties should be placed in the recovery position (*see page 34*) until help arrives.

4 If possible, obtain the bottle from which the poison came, or a sample of the poison itself.

5 If there is a residue of a caustic substance such as bleach or acid on the skin, this should be washed away with copious amounts of water.

# Alcohol Poisoning

Severe abuse of alcohol can cause serious poisoning and should be considered to be a life-threatening condition. Symptoms include:

- Vomiting
- Hot dry skin
- Heavy breathing
- Loss of consciousness

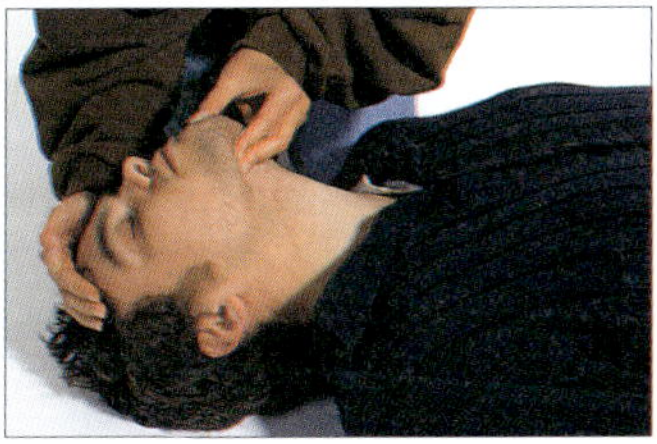

WHAT TO DO

1 Follow the ABC of resuscitation (*see page 21*) and be prepared to resuscitate (*see page 26*).

2 ☎ Call for an ambulance.

3 Place in the recovery position (*see page 34*), if the casualty is breathing. This is very important. Conscious victims may slip into unconsciousness and it is very common for victims of alcohol poisoning to die by choking on their own vomit.

4 Follow the ABC of resuscitation (*see page 21*) regularly, until help arrives.

# *Drug Overdose*

Every drug causes a different set of reactions and range of symptoms. In an overdose situation, any alarming behaviour or symptom patterns should be taken seriously. Hallucinations, intense drowsiness, collapse, loss of consciousness, nausea, vomiting and pain, seizures and cardiac arrest can all occur.

WHAT TO DO

1 ☎ Call for an ambulance immediately.

2 Treat as for poisoning (*see page 104*).

3 Follow the ABC of resuscitation (*see page 21*) and be prepared to resuscitate (*see page 26*).

4 If the casualty is breathing, place her in the recovery position.

NEVER give the victim of a drug overdose hot coffee or any other drinks which may accelerate the rate of absorption.

## Food Poisoning

Food poisoning is normally the result of inadequate hygiene or cooking. The two main types of bacteria which cause food poisoning are staphylococci and salmonella. Hepatitis A may also be passed on by food-handlers who have not washed properly.

> Any case of food poisoning which lasts for longer than 24 hours should be discussed with a doctor.

Symptoms include:

- Nausea, vomiting and diarrhoea.
- Pain in the abdomen and head.
- Fever (especially in the case of salmonella).
- Clinical shock (*see page 46*).

WHAT TO DO

1 Provide plenty of cool, fresh (or cooled boiled) water.

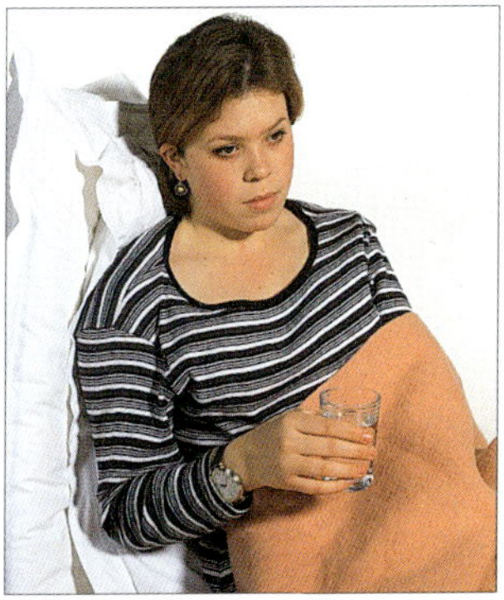

> To avoid the risk of dehydration, fluids should be drunk constantly while there is vomiting and diarrhoea. Suck ice cubes made of previously boiled water if vomiting makes it impossible to keep down fluids.
>
> Avoid milky drinks and anything which is acidic such as fruit juices.

# SMOKE INHALATION

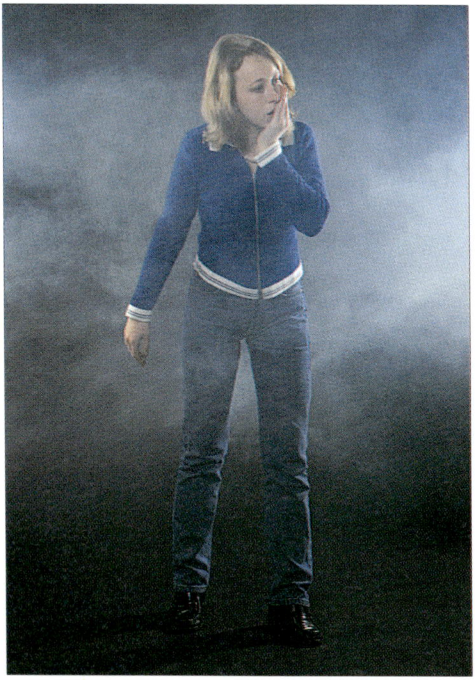

Smoke inhalation is most dangerous because of poisonous gases, which may kill, or irritate and even close the airway. The fire will draw on the oxygen in the immediate area, leading to suffocation.

NEVER risk your own life by entering a fume or smoke-filled area. Call the emergency services if you cannot safely remove the casualty from the source of the smoke.

Remember that the airway may be burned (*see page 51*) and may become obstructed due to inflammation, so it is important to monitor the casualty until the emergency services arrive.

Smoke may be poisonous, so get the casualty away from the area as soon as possible, without putting yourself at risk.

WHAT TO DO

**If conscious**

1 ☎ Call for an ambulance.

2 Treat any burns (*see page 49*) or injuries.

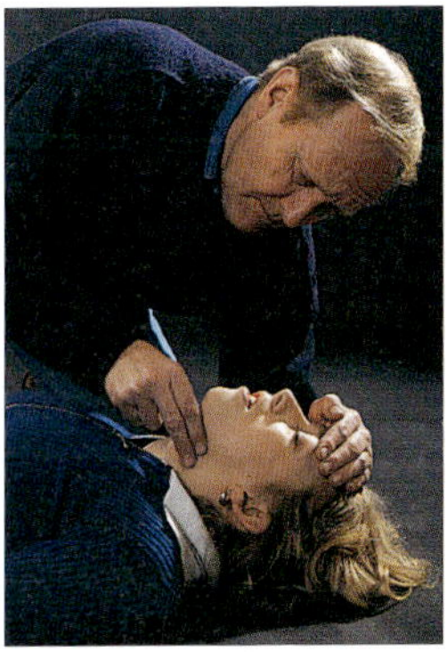

3 Check breathing and circulation regularly (*see page 22*) and be prepared to perform CPR (*see page 30*) if necessary.

**If unconscious**

1 ☎ Call for an ambulance.

2 Follow the ABC of resuscitation (*see page 21*) and be prepared to resuscitate (*see page 26*).

3 If the unconscious casualty is breathing, place her in the recovery position (*see page 34*) until help arrives.

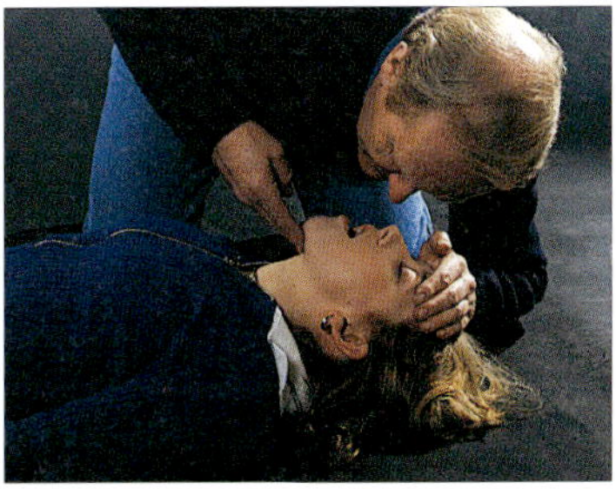

A conscious casualty may be given oxygen if it is available, but do not offer it unless you are trained in its use.

# STRANGULATION

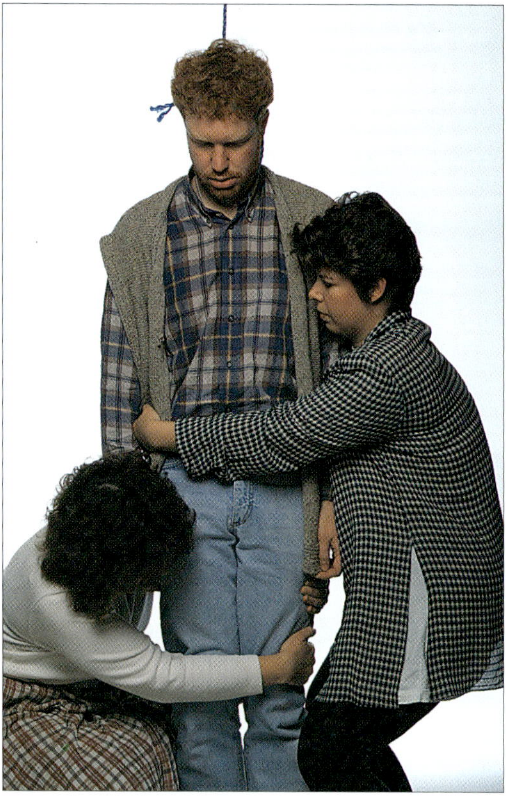

Strangulation is the constriction of the arteries and airway in the neck which will cause unconsciousness and death due to a lack of oxygen to the lungs and an inadequate supply of blood to the brain. Strangulation may be accidental or deliberate. If foul play is suspected do not move anything which could provide the police with evidence.

Strangulation may also be caused by hanging, which can result in a broken neck. Exercise extreme caution if strangulation is the result of hanging.

Signs of strangulation may include the presence of anything which has been used to constrict the neck, hoarse, laboured breathing, blueness around the mouth and perhaps the whole face, and bulging veins or eyes.

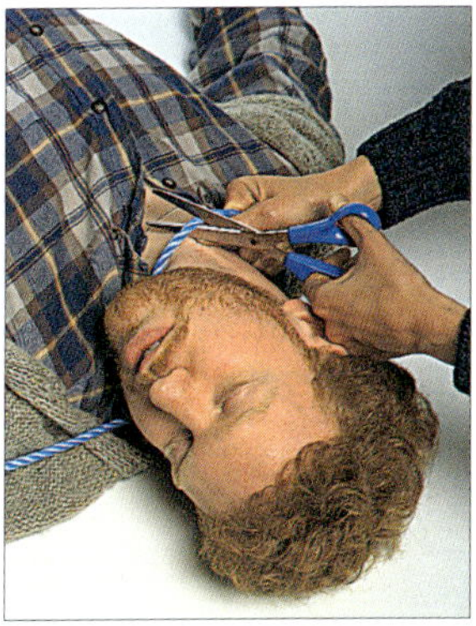

WHAT TO DO

1 Remove the constriction from around the neck by lifting the casualty carefully so that the weight is not on the neck. Cut the constriction rather than waste time trying to undo a knot.

2 ☎ Call for the emergency services.

**If conscious**

1 Keep the casualty calm until help arrives.

**If unconscious**

1 Immediately follow the ABC of resuscitation (*see page 21*) and be prepared to resuscitate (*see page 26*).

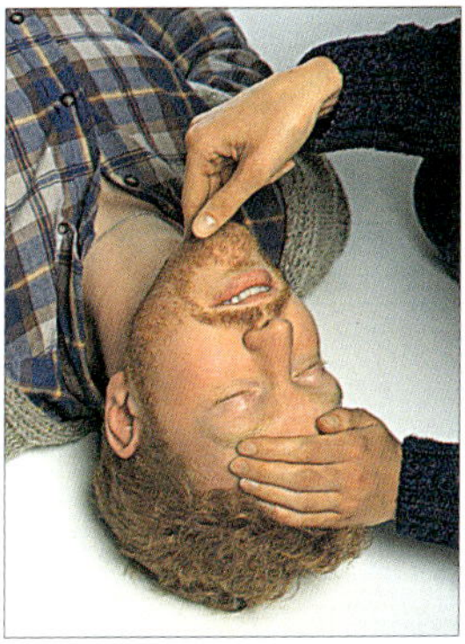

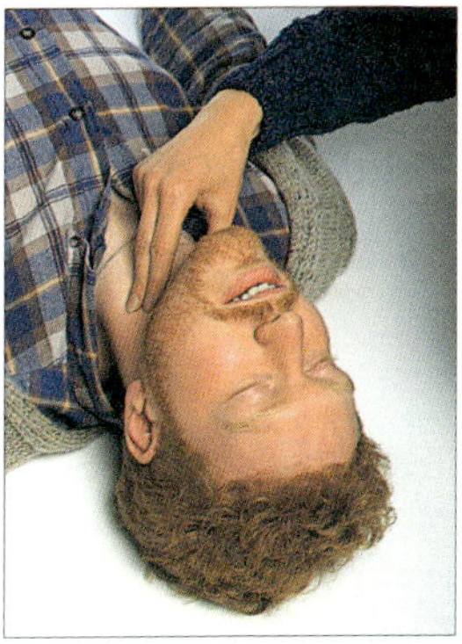

2 If the unconscious casualty is breathing, place in the recovery position (*see page 34*).

# STROKE

Stroke occurs when something causes a sudden interference in the blood supply to the brain. It is normally the result of a blood clot or a burst artery.

A casualty who is suffering a stroke may experience dizziness and occasionally confusion. The casualty may start to dribble or to show signs of paralysis or weakness on one side of the body. Unconsciousness may result. Certain types of stroke may cause a sudden blindingly painful headache, but these are relatively uncommon.

DO NOT give a stroke casualty anything to eat or drink.

## WHAT TO DO

1 ☎ Call for an ambulance.

**If conscious**

1 Lay the casualty down with his shoulders raised slightly. Ensure that he is comfortable and tilt his head to one side so that any saliva or vomit will drain away.

**If unconscious**

1 Immediately follow the ABC of resuscitation (*see page 21*) and be prepared to resuscitate (*see page 26*).

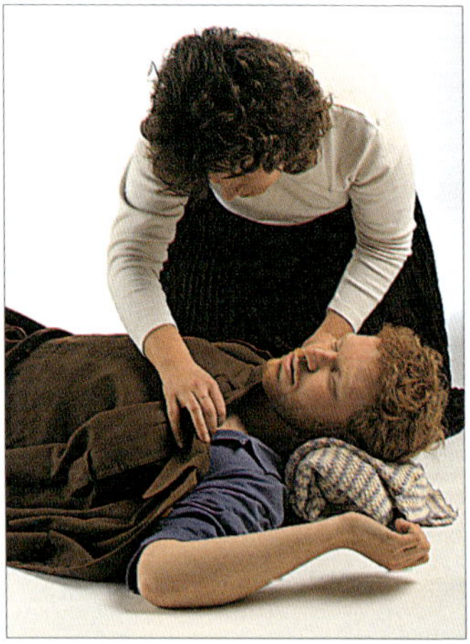

2 If the unconscious casualty is breathing, place him in the recovery position (*see page 34*).

# MISCELLANEOUS CONDITIONS

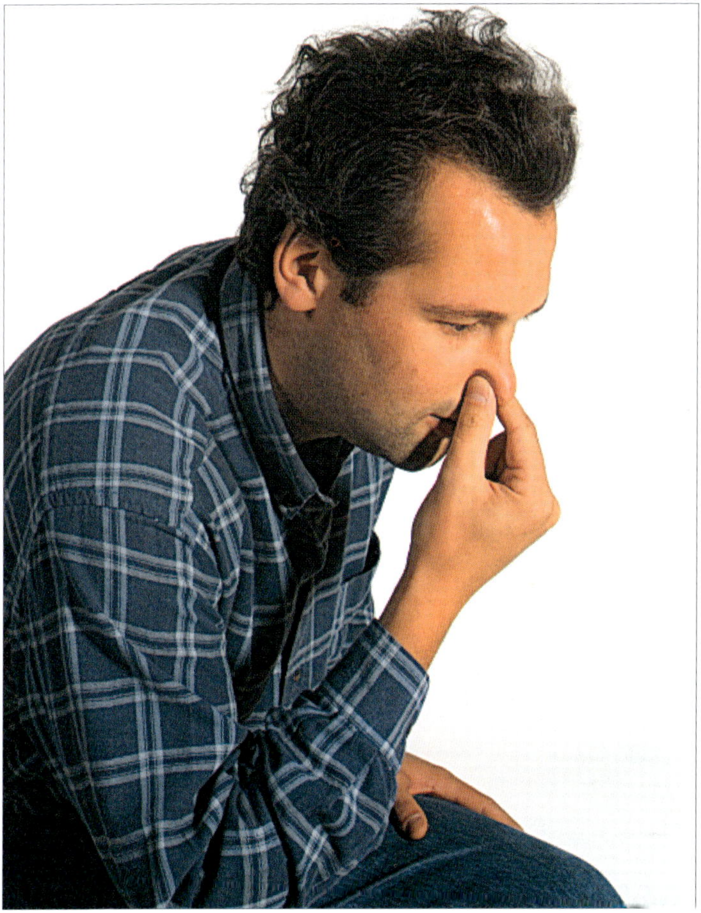

# BITES AND STINGS

## *Animal Bites*

Bites are potentially dangerous for two reasons: one, because the teeth of animals carry bacteria which can be thrust deep into tissues by the force of a bite, causing infection; and two, because they can be deep enough to damage tissue and occasionally to break bones. Some animals carry rabies, which is extremely serious. This condition is not found in the UK at present, but can be contracted while abroad, or from an animal smuggled in from a country abroad. If you suspect rabies, seek emergency medical attention.

## *Serious Wounds*

WHAT TO DO

1 Make the casualty comfortable and ensure that the injured part is elevated. Apply direct pressure to the wound using a sterile or very clean pad.

2 Bandage the pad into place.

3 Seek medical advice.

## *Shallow Wounds*

WHAT TO DO

1 Wash the wound carefully with soap and water. Dry gently and cover with a sterile pad or dressing.

2 Seek medical attention.

> Human bites can be as dangerous as animal bites for they can crush the tissues and cause infection.

## *Stings*

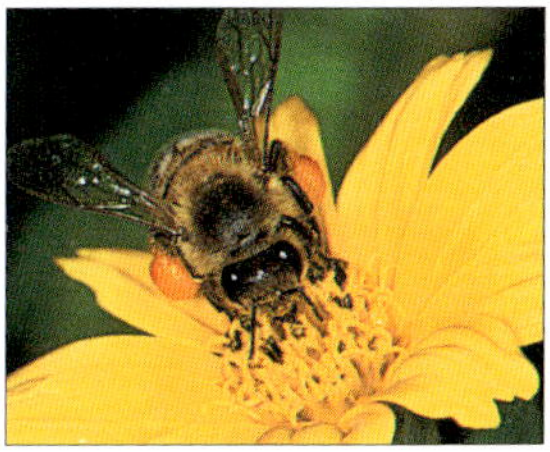

Stings from a bee, wasp or hornet are not usually dangerous unless the casualty suffers from an allergy to them. Multiple stings or stings in the mouth are obviously more serious and should be treated in a hospital. Stings in the throat or ears should also be treated immediately in hospital.

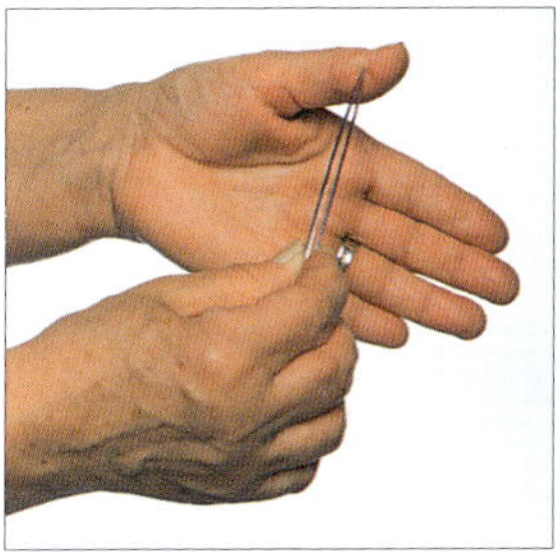

WHAT TO DO

1 With tweezers or two pins, remove the sting and rinse the area carefully.

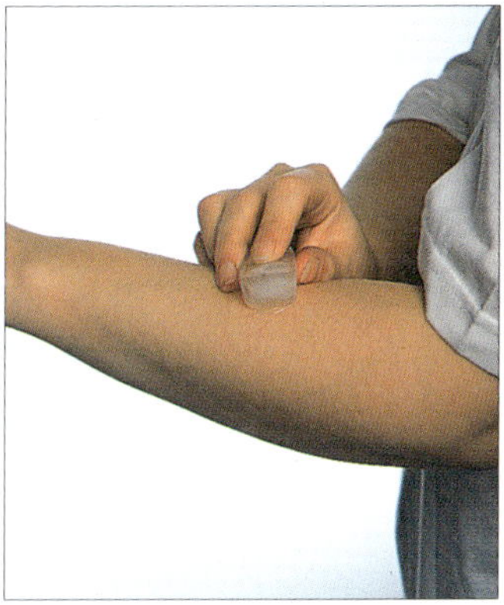

2 Apply a cold compress (*see page 134*) or an ice cube to ease the pain and reduce swelling.

3 ☎ If there are any signs of acute allergic reaction (*see page 54*), call for an ambulance.

4 If pain and swelling are persistent, seek medical advice.

# *Jellyfish stings*

Jellyfish, Portuguese men-of-war and other sea creatures can cause enormously painful stings, but most do not present a serious risk unless the stings are multiple. There is a small risk of a severe allergic reaction (*see page 54*).

WHAT TO DO

1 Pour alcohol or vinegar over the wound for a few moments. This may reduce further irritation.

2 Make a paste with equal proportions of bicarbonate of soda and water, and apply to the site of the stings.

☎ If the casualty has difficulty breathing, place in the recovery position (*see page 34*), call for an ambulance and follow the ABC of resuscitation (*see page 21*) very carefully.

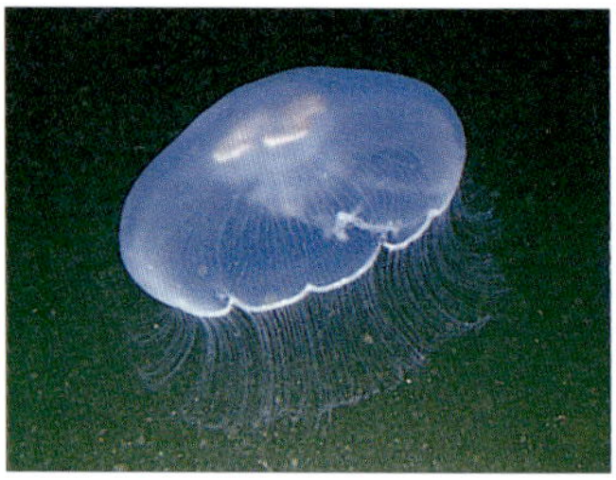

Jellyfish

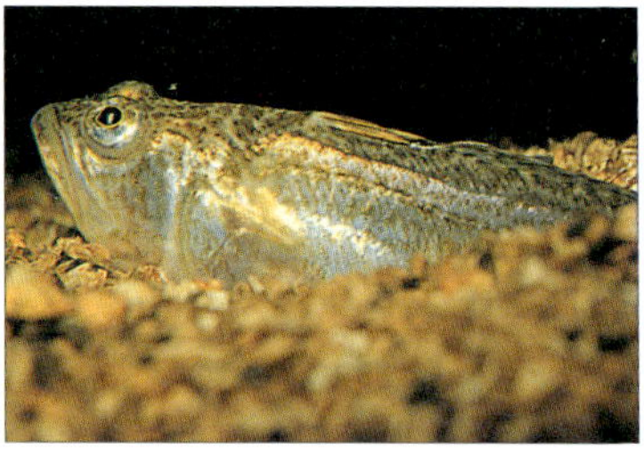

Weaver fish

# DIARRHOEA AND VOMITING

When diarrhoea and vomiting occur together they are usually the result of food poisoning, contaminated water or illness like viral gastro-enteritis. Consult your doctor if any case of vomiting or diarrhoea lasts for more than 24 hours.

> If you suspect food poisoning, seek advice from your doctor.

Diarrhoea and vomiting, particularly together, may cause dehydration, which is particularly dangerous in the very young and very old.

WHAT TO DO

1 Offer small sips of cooled, boiled water. If this does not stay down, suggest sucking an ice cube.

2 Prepare a drink which will replace body salts and electrolytes. Packets can be obtained from your chemist. In an emergency, add 1 teaspoon of salt and 4 teaspoons of sugar to one litre (2 pints) of water or orange juice, and sip.

> Only very plain food should be eaten for 24–48 hours following a bout of vomiting and diarrhoea.

*(see* ***Food Poisoning****, page 107)*

# DISLOCATION OF JOINTS

A dislocation occurs when a joint is forced out of position and this usually causes damage to the surrounding ligaments and tendons. A fracture may result if there was sufficient force. Some people regularly suffer dislocations because of unusually weak or lax muscles and ligaments surrounding the joint.

Characteristics of a joint dislocation include:

- Abnormal appearance of the joint.
- Inability to move the joint.
- Severe pain, swelling and occasionally bruising at the site.

Finger and shoulder joints are most commonly dislocated, but dislocations can occur anywhere.

WHAT TO DO

1 Support the joint and the limb in a comfortable position and maintain it there with a sling or cushion.

2 Arrange for the casualty to be transported to hospital.

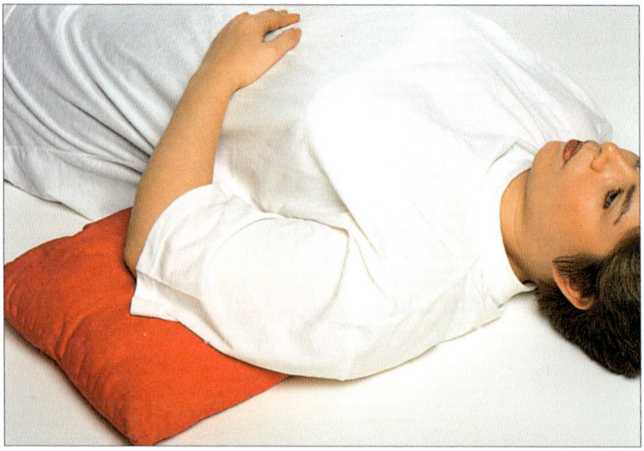

NEVER offer food or drink in case an operation requiring a general anaesthetic may be necessary.

NEVER attempt to pull the joint back into place.

# EAR CONDITIONS

Acute earache is most common in children, who are particularly susceptible to infections of the middle ear. Causes of earache include infection, a foreign object in the ear canal or a boil in the canal.

WHAT TO DO

1 Give Paracetamol or Ibuprofen.

NEVER give an aspirin to a child under the age of 12.

DO NOT give Ibuprofen to anyone allergic to aspirin.

If the pain does not settle or the casualty develops a discharge from the ear, or if fever develops, ask a doctor for advice.

## *Foreign Bodies in the Ear*

Children often push objects into their ears and they may block the ear canal causing temporary deafness and occasionally perforating the eardrum. Sharp objects may damage the ear canal and cause infection. Insects may also get into the ear canal and need to be removed.

WHAT TO DO

1 Seat the casualty so that she is comfortable and tilt her head so that the affected ear is upwards.

2 If you can see the object, pour water slowly into the ear canal so that it floats out.

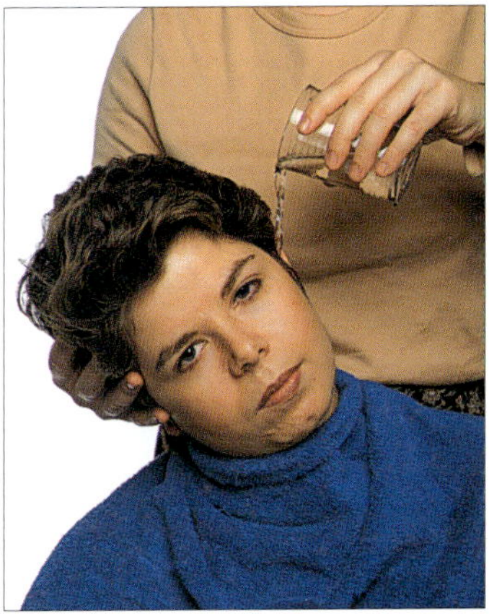

DO NOT attempt to remove the object if you cannot see it or if it is firmly lodged. Take the casualty to hospital.

# EYE INJURIES

Find out the cause of the injury. Establish whether it is the result of a chemical, a liquid or a foreign body in the eye.

WHAT TO DO

1 Seat the casualty or ask her to lie in a comfortable, well-lit area.

2 Wash your hands.

### Splashes in the eye

1 Ask her to look away, and pour copious amounts of water gently onto the conjunctiva (white of the eye). Encourage the casualty to move her eye around as you keep washing it.

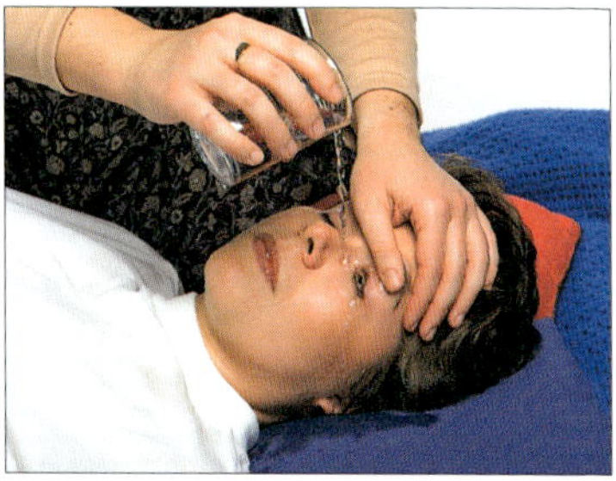

> If there is a harmful chemical in the eye, e.g. bleach, antifreeze, seek medical attention immediately.

### Foreign bodies in the eye

> NEVER attempt to remove anything that is embedded in the eye. In this case, both eyes should be covered and the casualty taken directly to hospital.

Treatment will depend upon the location of the foreign body:

- If the foreign body can be seen on the conjunctiva (white of the eye), gently wipe it off using a moist tissue or moist cotton wool bud.
- If the foreign body is on the cornea (the transparent covering over the iris and pupil), arrange for transportation to hospital.

# FAINTING

Fainting is a temporary loss of consciousness which is caused by a shortage of blood to the brain. In most cases, the cause is low blood pressure. A number of situations and conditions may cause fainting, including:

- Anxiety and fear
- Standing for long periods of time
- Intense or acute pain
- Extensive coughing
- Heat
- Pregnancy

Symptoms include a cold sweat, pale skin, dizziness and occasionally a ringing sound in the ears. These symptoms precede unconsciousness.

WHAT TO DO

1 Lay the casualty down with her feet on a level above her head – use a pile of books or clothing to prop them up.

2 Loosen any constrictive clothing.

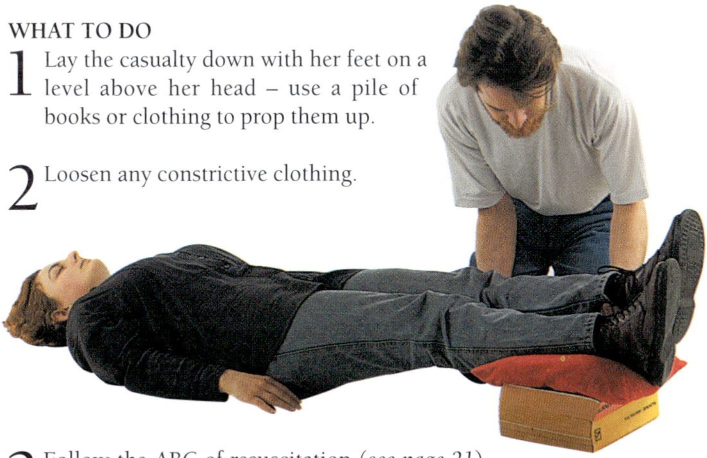

3 Follow the ABC of resuscitation (*see page 21*) and be prepared to resuscitate.

☎ The cause of the collapse may not be a simple faint. The casualty should recover consciousness within a few minutes. If she does not, call for an ambulance.

# NOSEBLEED AND FOREIGN BODIES IN THE NOSE

Nosebleeds are not usually serious, unless they are profuse. The lining of the nose is very sensitive and even blowing the nose heavily can rupture a tiny blood vessel and cause bleeding.

WHAT TO DO

1 Seat the casualty so he is comfortable and ask him to lean forward. He should pinch his nostrils together with his thumb and finger, applying firm, even pressure.

2 He should maintain this pressure for at least 10 minutes without raising his head.

> If the casualty experiences bleeding into the mouth, ask him to spit it out.

3 After 10 minutes, ask him to release the pressure very slowly and then carefully clean around the nose.

4 The nose should not be blown for the next 4 to 5 hours.

> If the bleeding does not stop, repeat steps 1–3. If this does not help, take the casualty to hospital.
>
> DO NOT put cotton-wool, etc. up the nose to make it stop.

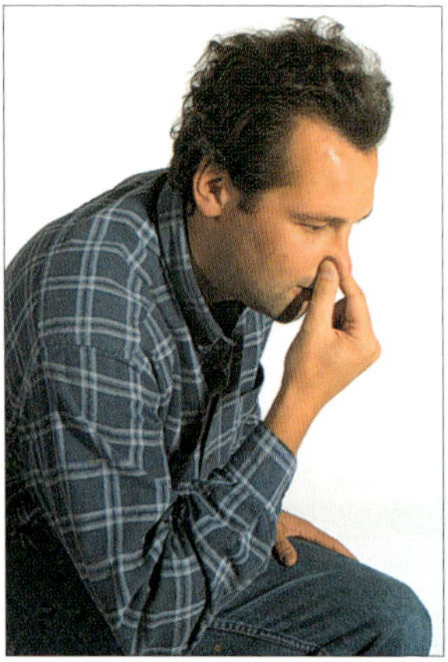

## *Foreign Bodies in the Nose*

A foreign body in the nose may be quite serious if the sensitive tissues and mucous membranes become damaged and infected. Some blockages are quite severe and will require surgery to loosen them.

DO NOT try to remove a foreign body which cannot be seen from the nose. You may push it in further or cause further damage.

Foreign bodies which can just be seen may be expelled by holding shut the other nostril and blowing hard through the nose. If it is blown to just inside the nostril, it may safely be removed with tweezers. This is the only case in which attempts should be made to remove the object.

WHAT TO DO

1 Keep the casualty calm and encourage him to breathe through his mouth. If he begins to panic, lay him down.

2 Take the casualty to hospital.

# SPLINTERS

A splinter is a small foreign body which has become lodged in the skin. Splinters are not serious, but they do present a risk of infection so they should be removed and the area cleaned as soon as possible.

## *Splinters with an end protruding*

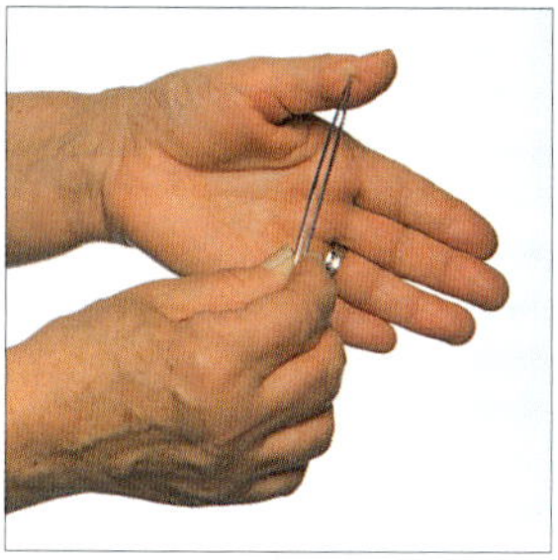

WHAT TO DO

1 Use tweezers to gently loosen and remove the splinter.

2 Wash the area carefully with soap and water and if there is bleeding, apply a plaster.

## *Splinters with no end protruding*

WHAT TO DO

1 Heat a thin needle or safety pin with a lighter or a match until it becomes hot. Allow it to cool slightly.

2 Gently ease one end of the splinter with the tip of the needle and catch the end with tweezers.

3 Wash the area carefully with soap and water and if there is bleeding, apply a plaster.

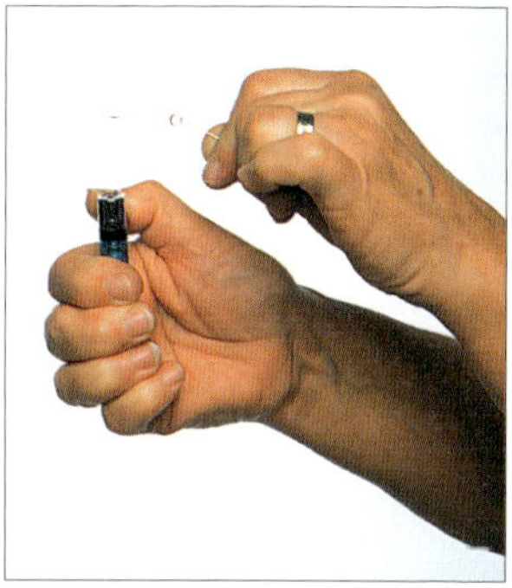

If you are unable to remove the splinter, see a doctor.

Glass splinters may splinter further, so be very gentle when using tweezers.

# SPRAINS AND STRAINS

A sprain can occur in any part of the body where there is a joint. A sprain is a ligament injury, and is usually the result of a wrench to the joint itself, which causes injury or tearing to the surrounding tissues. A strain is less serious than a sprain, and usually does not involve any tearing of the tissues.

Strains and sprains may be characterised by swelling, bruising and pain, and there is a simple procedure to follow. Remember RICE, which is:

R Rest the injured part.
I Ice is applied as a compress to the area. Cold water will do.
C Compress the immediate area.
E Elevate the injured part.

WHAT TO DO

1 Follow the RICE procedure by making the casualty comfortable, and ensuring that the injured part is resting on a cushion or some other form of support.

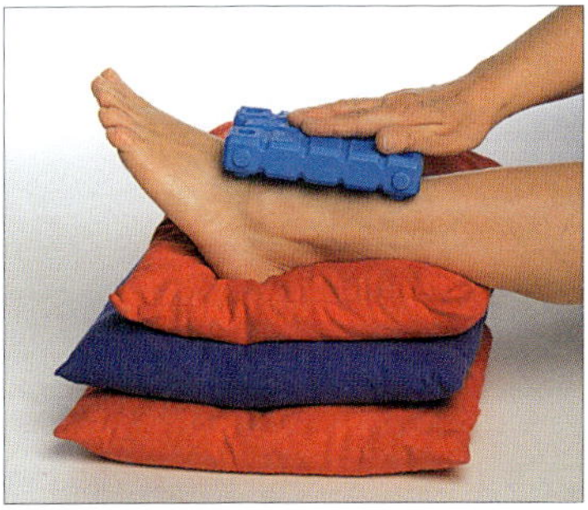

2 Cooling the area will prevent further swelling. It will also reduce pain and bruising.

3 Wrap a bandage (*see page 135*) or some cotton wool around the affected limb, compressing it so that it is held firmly.

4 Elevate the limb to prevent swelling.

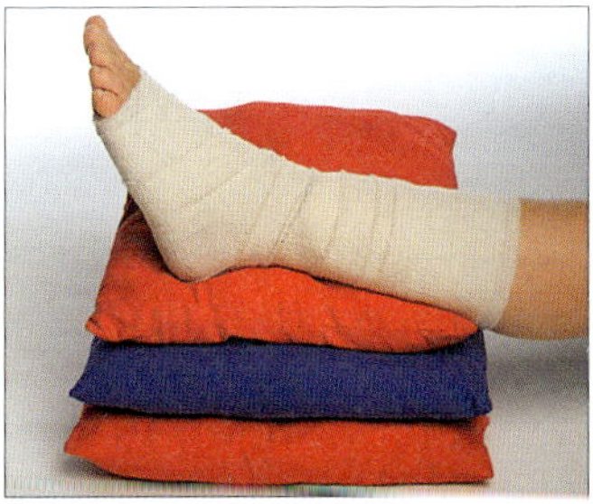

# SUNBURN

Sunburn is the result of overexposure to the ultraviolet rays of the sun, or a sun lamp. Sunburn is normally superficial, characterised by redness, some swelling and pain. More severe cases will blister and may be accompanied by heatstroke. Some people are more sensitive to the sun than others.

WHAT TO DO

1 Remove the casualty from the sun – indoors, if possible, since the rays of the sun can enter even shaded areas causing further damage.

2 Cool the skin by pouring cold water over the affected areas, or by very gently sponging the skin. A cool bath might be helpful.

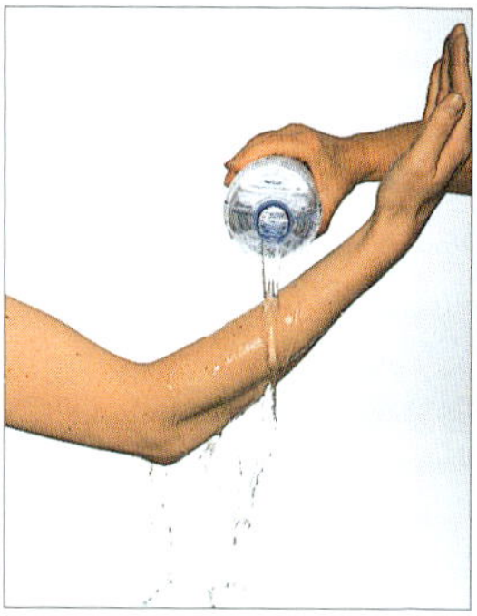

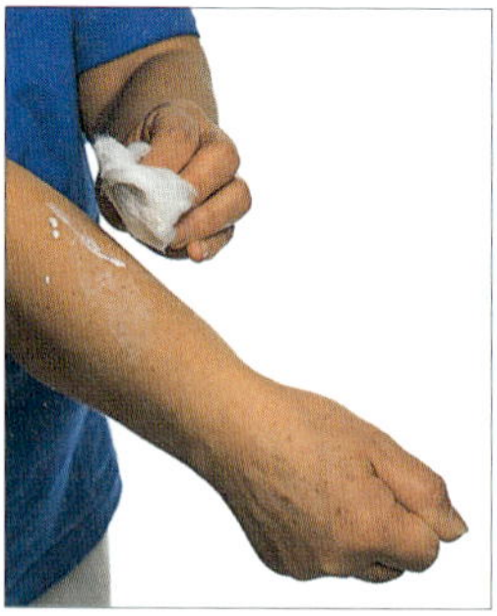

Avoid a sudden very cold bath.

3 Offer sips of cold water and dress the skin with a soothing lotion like aloe or calamine.

4 Watch for signs of blistering, which should be brought to the attention of a doctor.

# TEMPERATURE (HIGH)

There are a number of causes for high temperature, some more serious than others. The great majority are caused by infection or overheating.

Most fevers can be controlled at home with Paracetamol and sponging with lukewarm water, but if the temperature rises above 40°C (102°F) ring your doctor. Fevers in small children can cause febrile convulsions (*see page 74*).

WHAT TO DO

1 Ensure that the casualty is comfortable and has one blanket only.

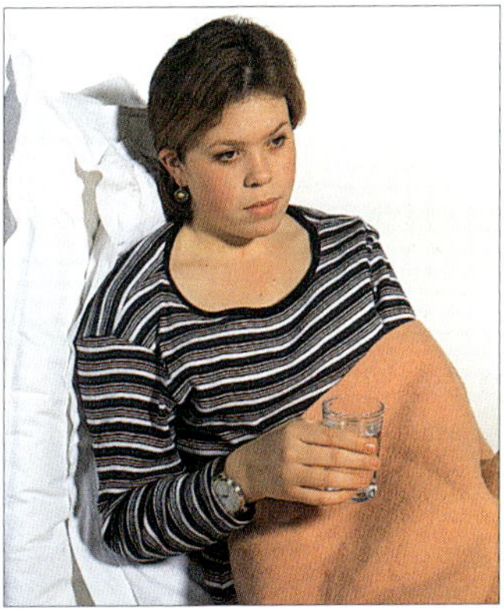

2 Offer plenty of cool fluids.

3 Paracetamol or aspirin may be given to adults to bring down the fever.

NEVER give aspirin to a child under the age of 12.

4 Sponge the casualty with lukewarm water or, if possible, put her in a lukewarm bath.

5 ☎ If the fever begins to cause convulsions, treat for convulsions (*see page 74*), and call for a doctor or ambulance.

CHILDREN

1. Children should be sponged with lukewarm water or placed in a tepid bath.
2. Offer paracetamol syrup in the correct dosage. Do not give aspirin.
3. Any temperature that rises to over 40°C (102°F) should be reported to a doctor.

# TOOTHACHE AND KNOCKED-OUT TEETH

## *Toothache*

Toothache is normally the result of decay, gum disease or an abscess. Pain from these can vary, but in all cases should be seen by a dentist. Some toothache may be the result of 'referred pain' from other conditions like sinusitis, ear infections or problems with the jaw.

WHAT TO DO

1 Arrange to see a dentist.

2 Take painkillers like Paracetamol or Ibuprofen.

3 Make the casualty comfortable until dental treatment is available. It may help to keep the upper body elevated.

Avoid eating or drinking anything that aggravates the pain, e.g. foods that are too hot, cold, spicy or hard.

Do-it-yourself dental first aid kits are available in shops. These may be used while awaiting treatment.

## *Knocked-out Teeth*

Teeth that have been knocked out of their sockets can often be successfully implanted again.

WHAT TO DO

1 Place the tooth in the side of the mouth or in a glass of milk to stop it drying out.

2 Seek emergency treatment with a dentist or hospital.

DO NOT try to reimplant the tooth yourself. See a dentist as soon as possible to maximise the chance of successful reimplantation.

If you need to wash the tooth, gently rinse it in cold water, holding it by the crown, not the roots.

## *Gum and Socket Bleeding*

Bleeding which happens every time you brush your teeth is probably caused by gum disease, so arrange a dental check up to seek advice and treatment. Unusual bleeding soon after you've had a tooth out is probably from the socket and is more urgent.

WHAT TO DO

1 Roll up gauze or a small piece of clean fabric and place it over the entrance to the socket.

2 Press down on the pad to apply pressure to the socket and to stop the bleeding.

3 Do this for 10 minutes and then remove the pad carefully to see if the bleeding has stopped, taking care not to disturb the clot if you can. If it is still bleeding, repeat steps 1 and 2 and check again.

4 Bleeding usually stops after two or three attempts at this. If it doesn't, seek dental or medical advice immediately.

# TRAVEL SICKNESS

Some people are more susceptible to travel sickness (also called motion sickness) than others. It is caused by continuous motion and is characterised by the following symptoms:

- Harsh breathing.
- Nausea.
- Excess salivation.
- Abdominal cramps and occasionally diarrhoea.
- Pale, sweating skin.
- Vomiting and dizziness.
- Yawning.
- Headache and overwhelming fatigue.

WHAT TO DO

1 Fresh air will help. Seat the casualty outside, or with the window rolled down, with his head tilted backwards.

2 On a boat ask the casualty to fix his eyes on a point on the horizon and breathe deeply.

3 On an aeroplane, turn the cool air on the casualty's face, tilt his head back and ask him to breathe deeply.

4 Some people find seabands, slim bands worn on the wrist which press against acupressure points, useful for long journeys. These can be purchased in advance at a chemist.

DO NOT drink alcohol or eat anything fatty. Before a long or bumpy journey, eat a small quantity of easily digested food.

# DRESSINGS, BANDAGES AND HANDLING

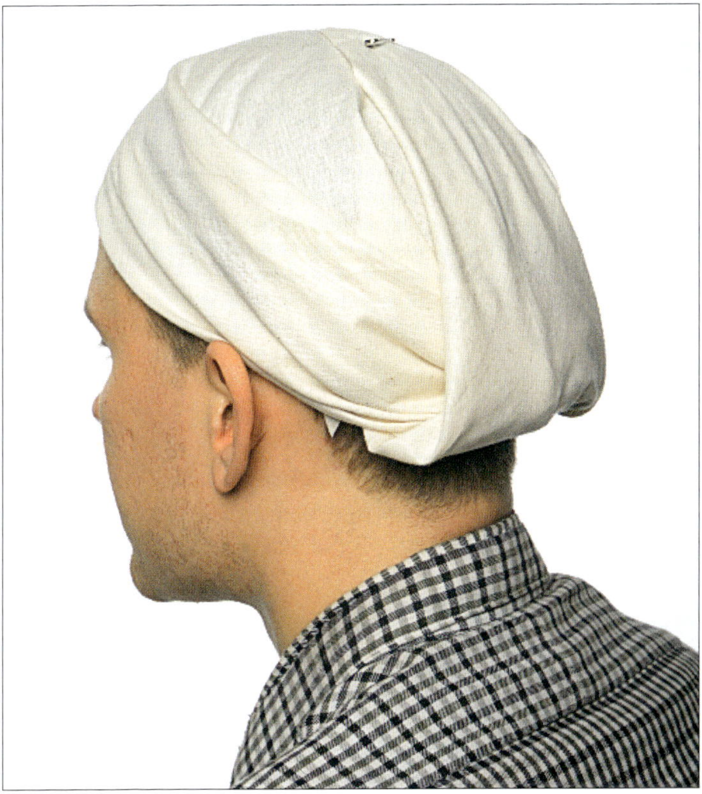

# DRESSINGS

Dressings are used to prevent germs entering the bloodstream through a wound, and to help staunch the flow of blood, allowing it to clot. There are many types of dressing and they will be applied according to the nature of the wound. Dressings should always be sterile and made of a fabric which will 'breathe' or allow air at the wound to encourage healing and to allow sweat to evaporate. Any dressing that is allowed to get wet becomes a breeding ground for bacteria.

NEVER use fluffy material as a dressing because fibres will stick to the wound.

## Applying a Dressing

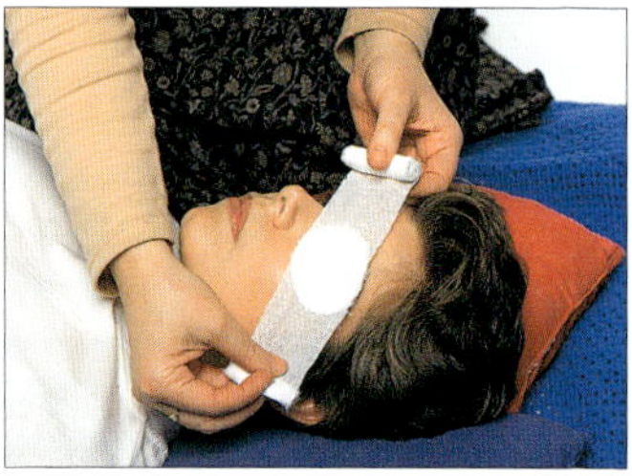

- Wash your hands carefully before applying a dressing.
- Clean the skin and the surrounding area gently before applying a dressing.
- All dressings should be about 2.5cm (1 in) larger all round than the wound they are to cover.
- Place the dressing directly on the wound.

DO NOT touch the wound or the part of the dressing that will be applied over it.

NEVER remove a dressing and start again, for any blood clot which has formed will be disturbed. If blood soaks through as you work, apply another dressing on top.

## Plasters

- Plasters should be held over the wound they are to cover.
- Remove the wrapping and pull back the strips over the adhesive.
- Press down the edges of the plaster over the wound.

## Sterile Pads

- Place the pad with the absorbent side on the wound and secure with a bandage, strapping or taping from the base of the injury up the limb itself.
- Tape the edge of the bandage with hypoallergenic tape.

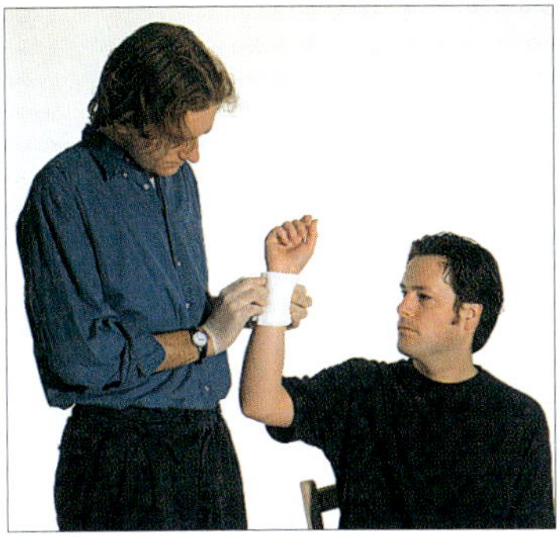

Some sterile pads come complete with a roller bandage attached (*see page 135*). In these cases, hold the bandage either side of the dressing and place the dressing on the wound.

- Pull the short end of the bandage tight, and then wrap the long end around the limb until the dressing is covered.
- Tie together the two ends of the bandage over the pad.

## Gauze Bandages

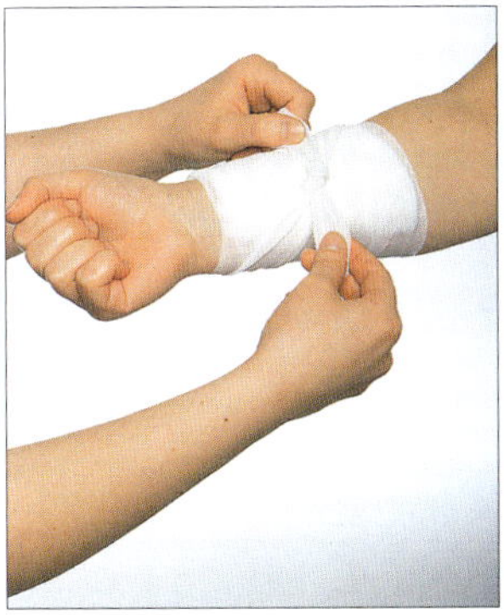

Gauze bandages do not usually have an adhesive side and they are usually used for large wounds which should only be lightly bandaged.

- Unwrap the gauze and place firmly on the wound.
- Cover the dressing with a pad of cotton wool, for absorbency.
- Bandage the dressing and the cotton wool in place with hypoallergenic tape or a bandage (*see page 132*).

## Improvised Dressings

In an emergency situation, you may not have access to prepared dressings. Any clean, preferably sterile, dry and non-fluffy fabric can be used as a dressing, and secured with a scarf or handkerchief that can be tied or pinned in place.

# COMPRESSES

A compress is applied to the body on a temporary basis, in order to heat or cool the affected area. Compresses are easily improvised, although you can purchase ready-made compresses that can be kept in your freezer (cold) or that radiate their own heat when activated (hot).

## *Cold*

The application of a cold compress chills areas of the tissues so that arterial circulation is closed down locally. This relieves swelling without interfering with the healing process. Cold also reduces the sensitivity of the nerves and therefore, pain. In general a compress should remain in place for about 30 minutes, but it may need to be changed every 10–12 minutes, as needed.

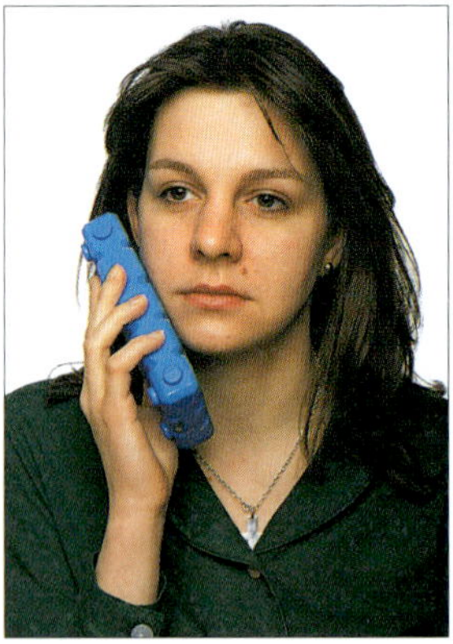

A cold compress may comprise:

- A towel, dipped in cold water and wrung nearly dry.
- Frozen peas, wrapped in a handkerchief or towel. These are particularly useful because unlike ice they mould to the body contours.
- A bag of ice cubes, mixed with salt to allow the ice to melt.

## *Hot*

A hot compress is used to relieve pain and muscle spasm, but because it increases the flow of blood to the area, blood clotting can be retarded. Hot compresses are for short-term relief only (10–15 minutes).

A hot compress may comprise:

- A hot-water bottle.
- A towel soaked in hand-hot water.

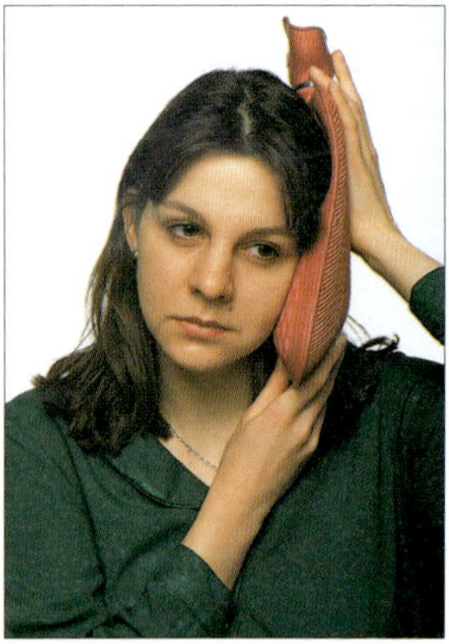

# BANDAGES

There are two main types of bandage: roller bandages and triangular bandages. There are also several types of bandage that are made of gauze and do not require fastenings, such as the tubular gauze bandages.

Bandages are used to apply pressure to a limb in order to:

- Hold the dressings in place.
- Prevent swelling.
- Support an injury.
- Prevent movement.

## *Applying a Bandage*

- Always make sure that the casualty is seated or lying comfortably.
- Stop if you are causing any pain.
- Always work from the injured side of a casualty.
- Make sure the injured limb is supported.
- When bandages are used to immobilise a fracture, tie knots on the uninjured side.
- Bandages must be firm but never so tight as to cut off circulation. Remember that injuries may cause swelling, so bandages should be checked frequently to ensure that they are not too tight.

## *Roller Bandages*

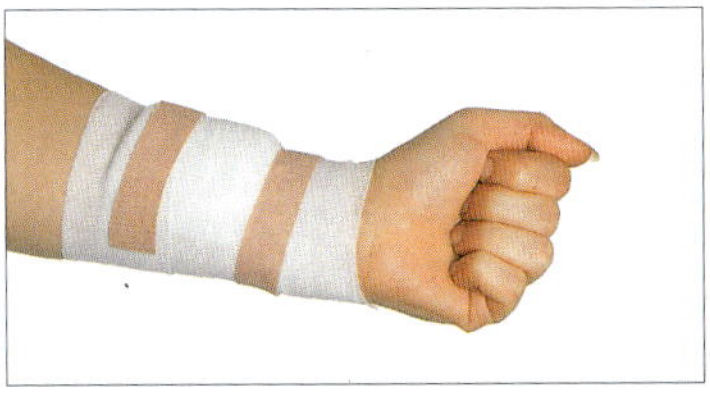

Roller bandages are usually made of cotton, gauze or linen and can be purchased in a roll, hence their name. There are different widths for various parts of the body:

| | |
|---|---|
| 2.5cm (1 in) | finger |
| 5cm (2 in) | hand |
| 5–6cm (2–2½ in) | arm |
| 7.5–9cm (3–3½ in) | leg |
| 10–15cm (4–6 in) | trunk |

## Spiral Bandaging

1 Support the injured limb and hold the bandage with one end at the top.

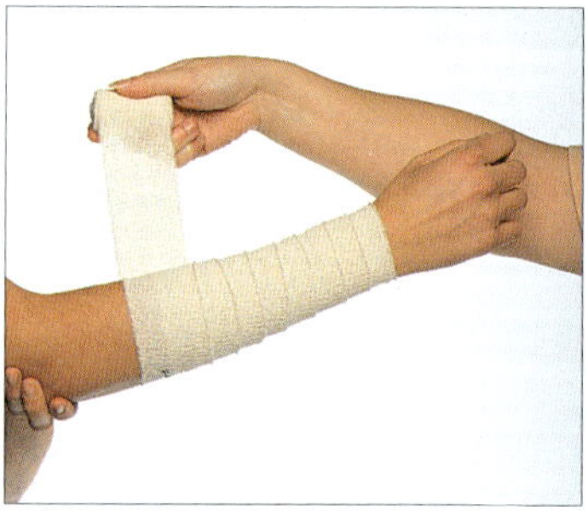

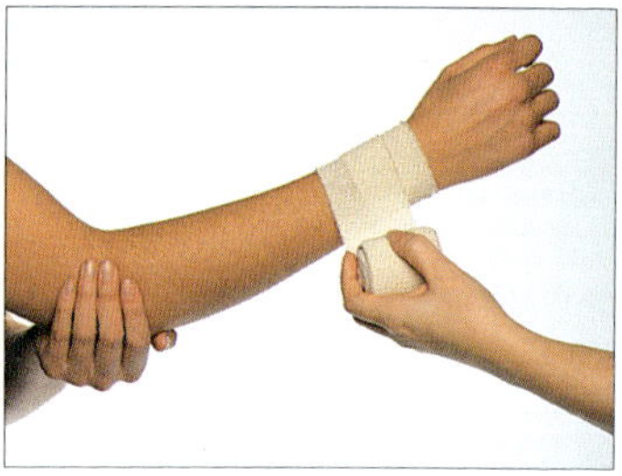

2 Wrap the bandage twice round that top end and begin to spiral the bandage up the limb, allowing each spiral to cover about half of the previous layer.

3 Towards the end of the bandage, spiral once or twice on top of the previous layer.

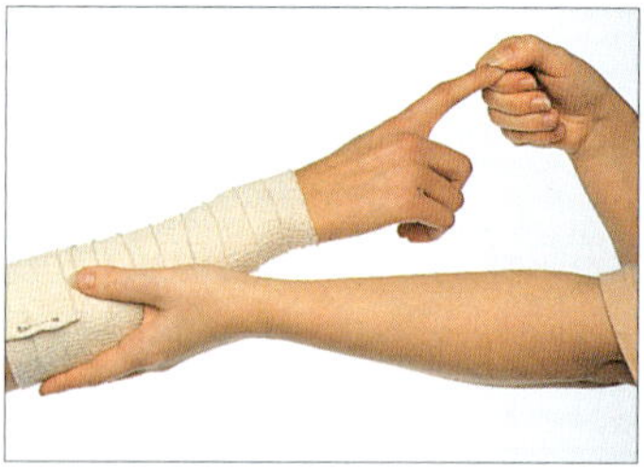

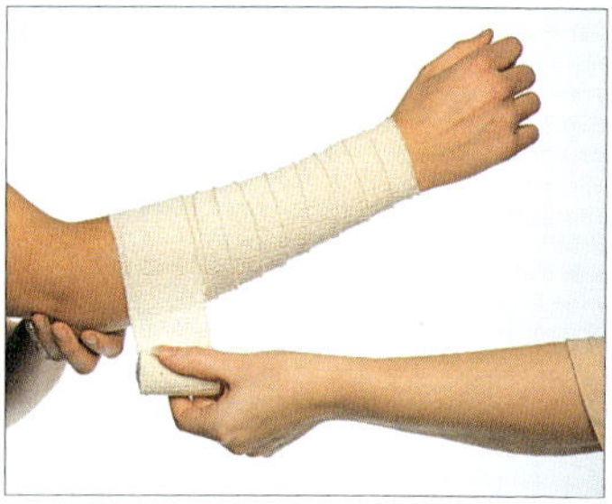

4 Check that the bandage is not too tight, and then secure (*see page 137*).

If the bandage is not long enough, add another one, wrapping several times over the end of the first with one end, and then continuing the spiral up the limb.

## *Securing a Bandage*

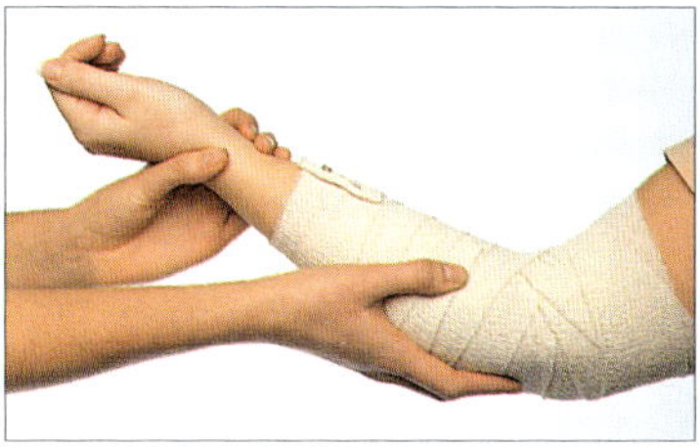

Some bandages come with pins or clips that hold one end against the body. Always secure a bandage on the uninjured side of a fracture, or on the gauze pad side of a wound.

Other forms of securing a bandage include:

- Safety pins.
- Adhesive tape.
- Tying (*see Reef Knot, page 147*).

TYING A BANDAGE

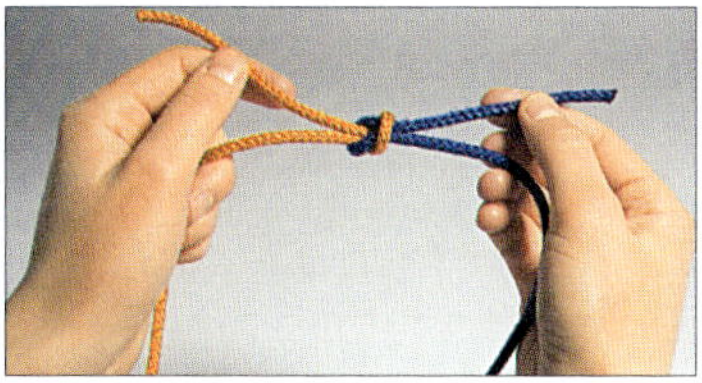

(Coloured cord has been used here for clarity.)

1. Leave enough of the bandage end free to tie and then slit the bandage down the centre until you have two lengths which are long enough to wrap around the limb.
2. Wrap one end in one direction and the other around the other side and tie them in a reef knot (*see page 147*).

## *Bandaging a Hand or Foot*

Use a roller bandage (*see page 135*) to hold a dressing in place or to support the wrist or ankle where there is a strain or sprain.

1 Support the injured limb. Put the bottom of the bandage on the inside of the wrist or ankle. Turn twice on top of the tail end.

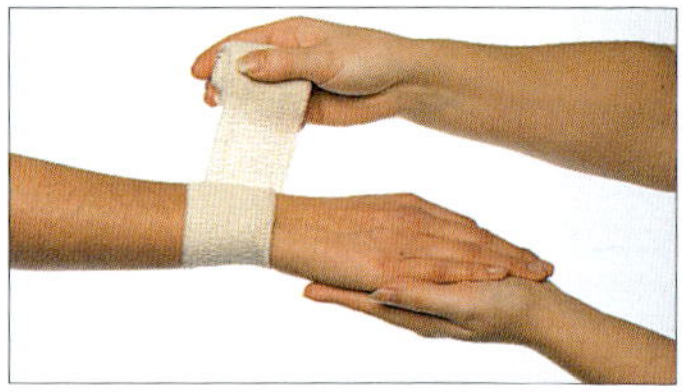

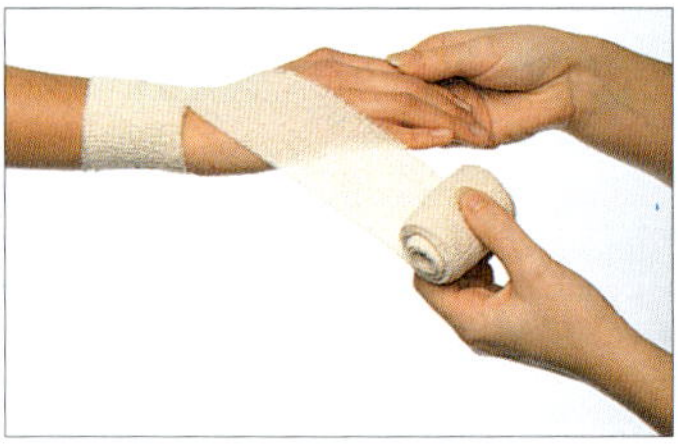

2 Wrap the bandage diagonally across the back of the casualty's hand, across the little finger and under the hand across the base of the fingers.

3 Wrap it diagonally across the back of the hand and wrap it several times around the wrist.

4 Carry the bandage up diagonally again, and repeat steps 2 and 3, working the bandage towards the wrist but keeping the thumb unbandaged.

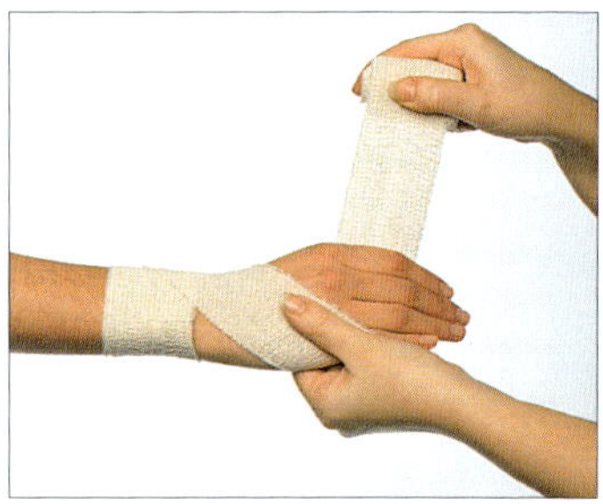

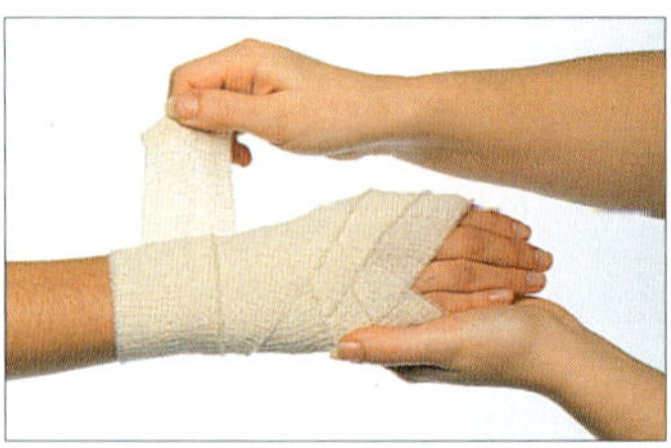

5 When the hand is entirely covered by the bandage, wrap it several times around the wrist and secure (*see page 137*).

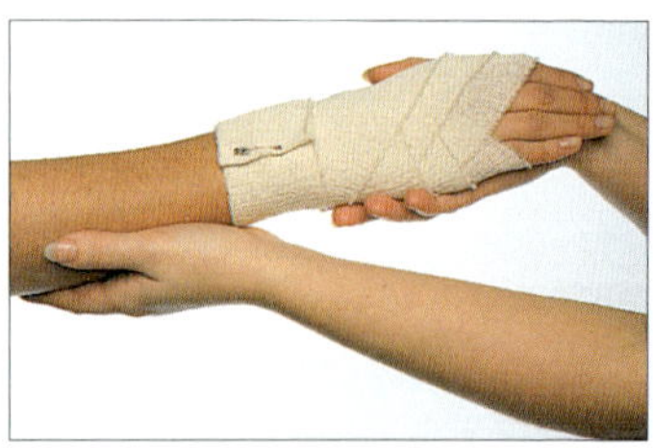

6 Check that the bandage is not too tight, and rebandage if there are signs that circulation is impeded. Use the same process for a foot.

## *Bandaging an Elbow or Knee*

Use a roller bandage (*see page 135*) for joint bandaging, either to hold a dressing in place or to support a strain or sprain. Suspected fractures of a joint should not be bandaged.

1 Support the injured limb so that it is partly bent.

DO NOT bend the limb if you suspect a fracture or if this movement causes any pain.

2 Put the bottom of the bandage on the inside of the elbow. Wrap it twice to cover the joint.

3 Holding the rolled end of the bandage, wrap it firmly around the joint, and then wrap it once around the upper arm, covering about half of the first layer.

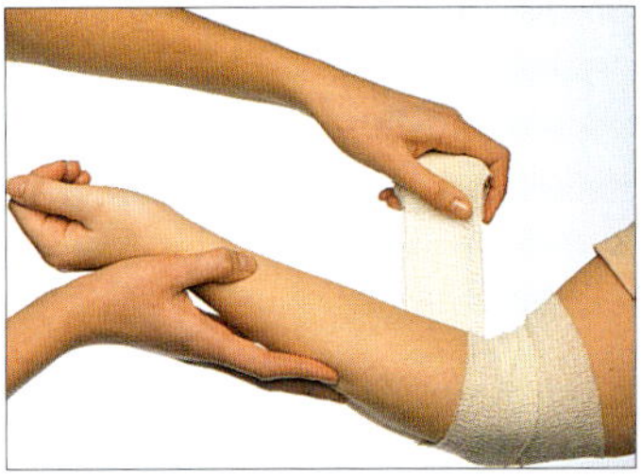

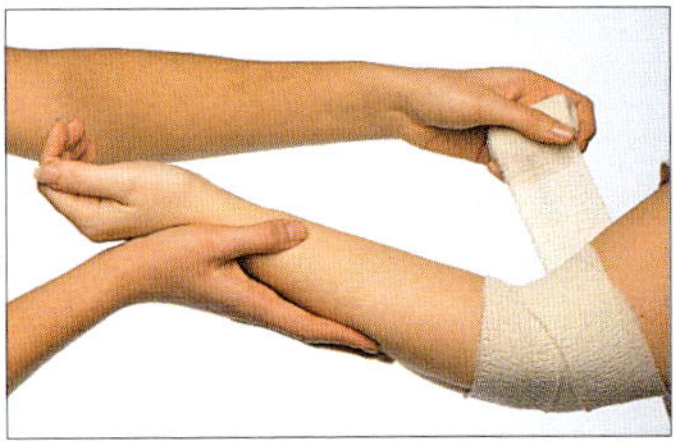

4 Bring the bandage under the joint and wrap it firmly around the bottom part of the elbow, again covering about half of the first layer.

5 Work your way up and down the arm until the bandage covers the joint and half of the upper and lower arm.

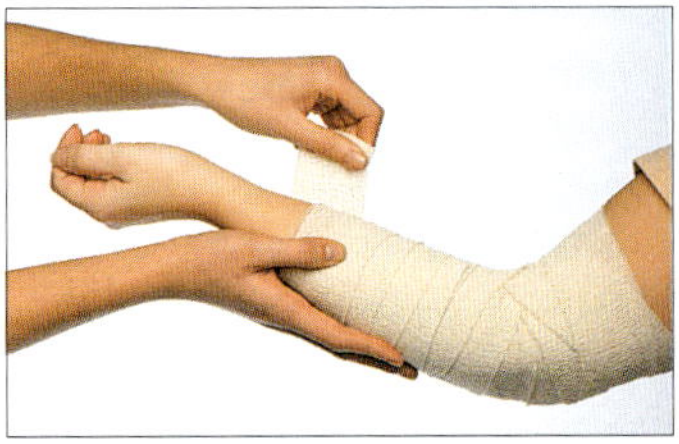

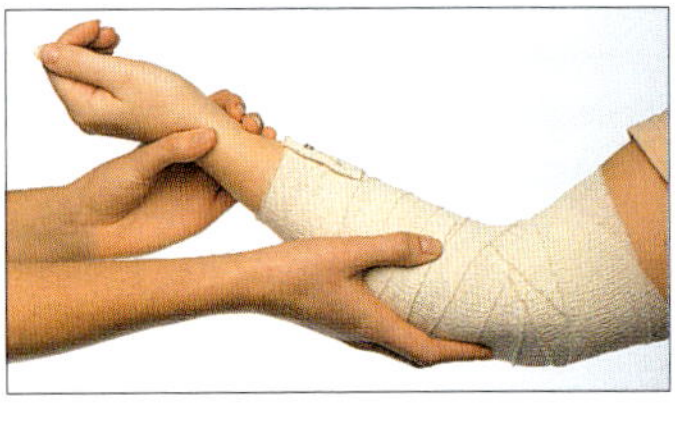

6 Secure the bandage (*see page 137*) and check that it is not too tight. Rebandage if there are signs that circulation is impeded. Use the same process for a knee.

## *Triangular Bandage*

A triangular bandage is normally used as a sling to support or protect a limb, but it may also be used:

- To secure dressings on the head, hand or foot.
- To make a broad or narrow bandage (*see below*).

SLINGS (*see page 145*)

### BROAD BANDAGES

Broad bandages are useful for the immobilisation and support of fractures, and for securing splints and large dressings.

1 Fold the base so that there is a thin hem line.

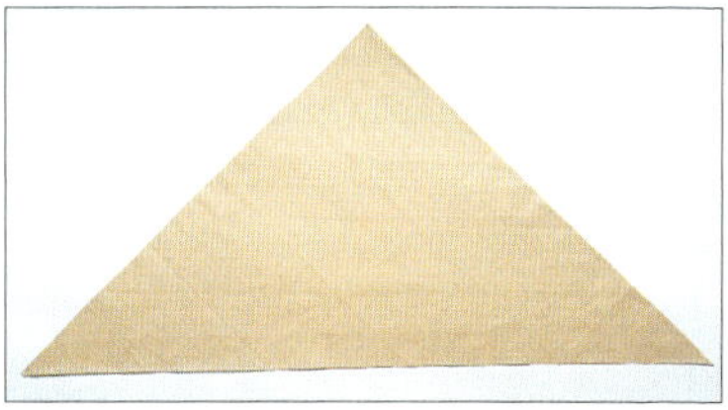

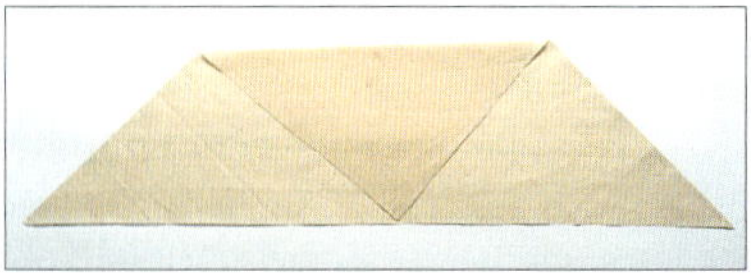

2 Fold the top point towards the base so that it touches the new hem line.

3 Fold the bandage in half again, in the same direction.

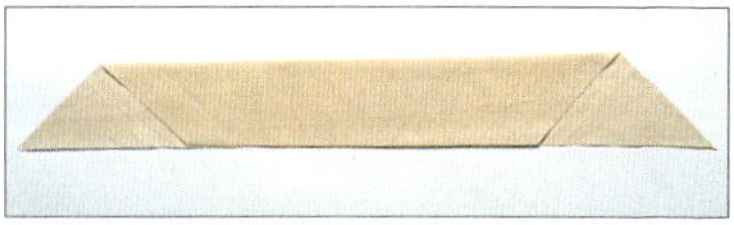

### NARROW BANDAGES

A narrow bandage is used to immobilise feet and ankles in the case of a fracture, and to secure dressings to the limbs, particularly those at the wrist or ankle joints.

1 Make a broad bandage (*see steps 1–3 above*).

2 Fold the bandage in half again.

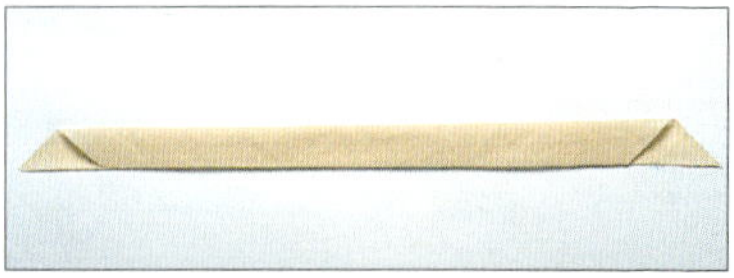

## Figure-of-eight Bandage

A figure-of-eight bandage is used to immobilise feet and ankles in the case of a fracture.

1 Find a narrow bandage and liberally pad both sides of the injured leg, taking special care between the limbs.

2 Feed the bandage under the hollows of the ankles so that there are even lengths on either side of the legs.

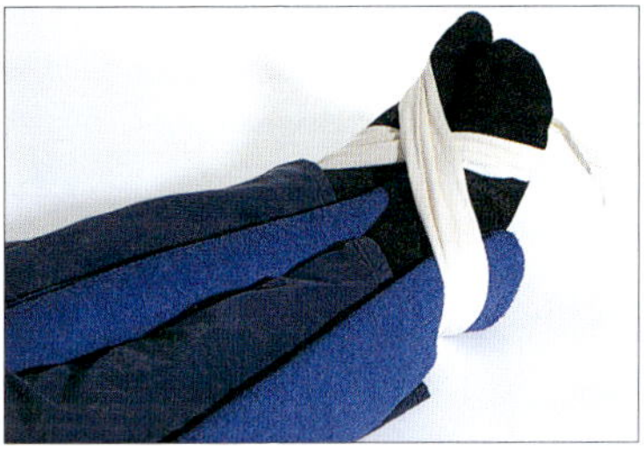

3 Cross the bandage above the ankles and then bring the ends down and tie them firmly under the soles of the feet using a reef knot (*see page 147*).

## Scalp Bandage

The scalp may be bandaged using a triangular bandage (*see page 140*) that has not been folded. Dressings may be held in place by a triangular bandage, but there will be insufficient pressure to staunch the blood so this method of bandaging is unsuitable when there is serious bleeding.

1 Place the bandage on the head of the casualty, with the hem across the forehead at the level of the eyebrows. The point should be hanging down the centre of the back.

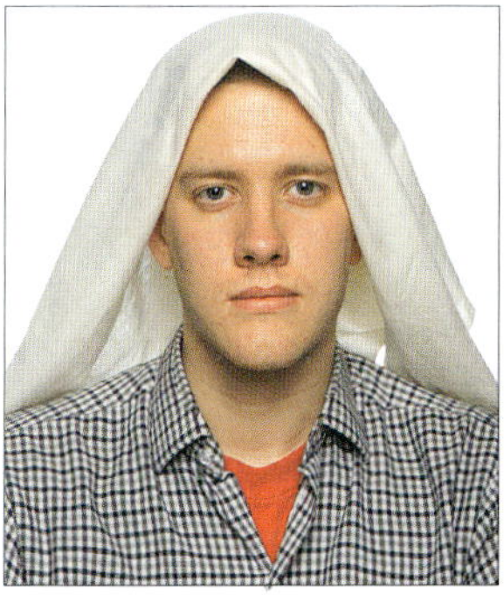

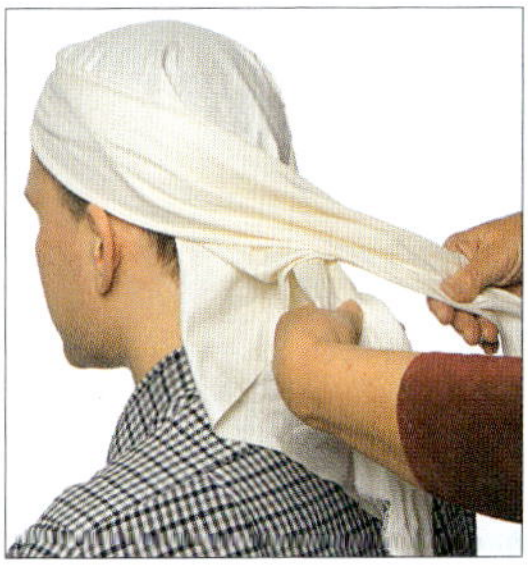

2 Take the two side points of the bandage round the back, lifting them above the ears.

3 Cross the two ends over the point of the bandage and carry them around the front of the head.

4 Fasten the two ends with a reef knot (*see page 147*).

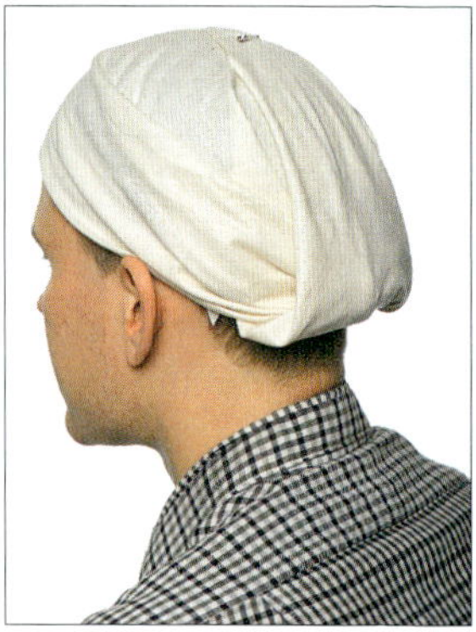

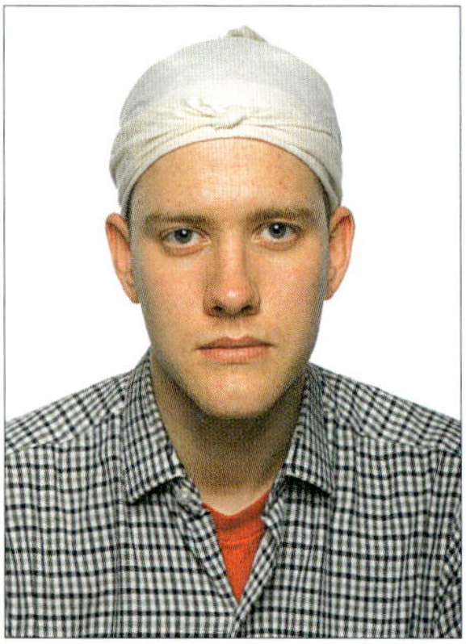

5 Gently pull down the point of the bandage until there is consistent pressure, and then gently secure it to the bandage on the top of the head.

## *Hand and Foot Bandages*

A triangular bandage is useful for securing a large dressing on hands and feet, although there will not be enough pressure to staunch any bleeding. This is most useful for large wounds which are too large for standard bandage procedures.

1 Place the hand palm down on the triangular bandage with the hem level with the base of the wrist and the point folded down over the back of the hand.

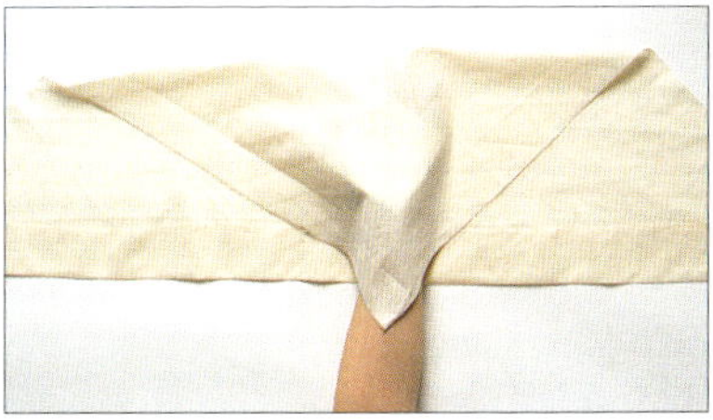

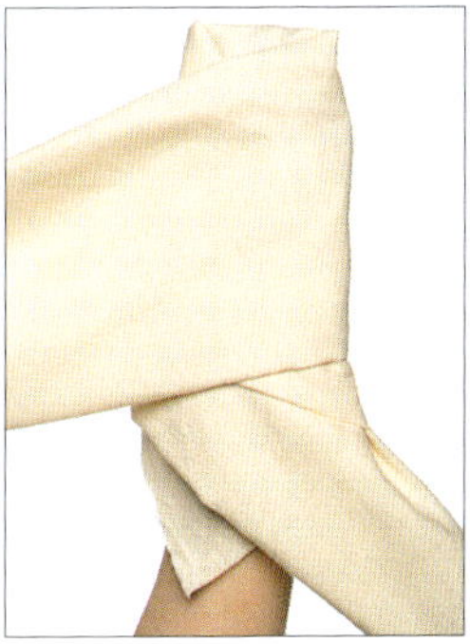

2 Make sure the dressing is firmly in place, and then cross the two ends of the bandage around the wrist, cross them again, and then tie them using a reef knot (*see page 147*).

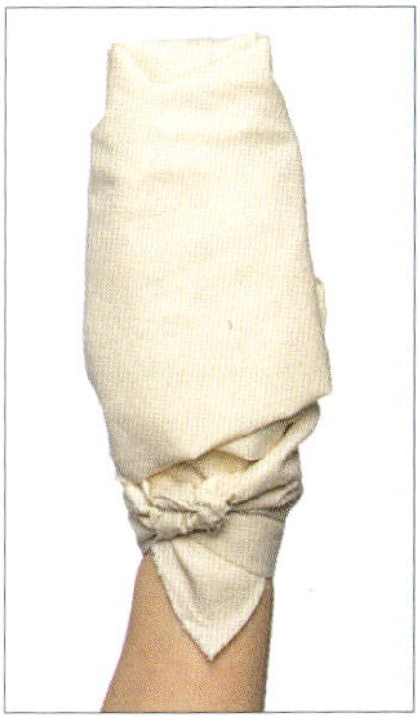

3 Pull down the point of the bandage to tighten it, but take care not to impede the circulation.

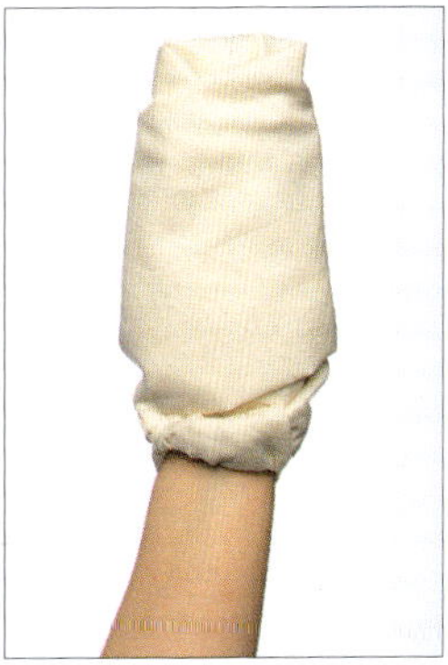

4 Pull the point up and over the knot, and then tuck it in beneath. Use the same process for a foot.

## Tubular Gauze Bandages

These bandages come in rolls and are cut to the correct length. They are suitable for holding dressings in position, but they will not exert enough pressure to staunch bleeding. Many tubular bandages come with an applicator, but this is not always the case. When used on the ankle, leg or arm, no fastening will be necessary.

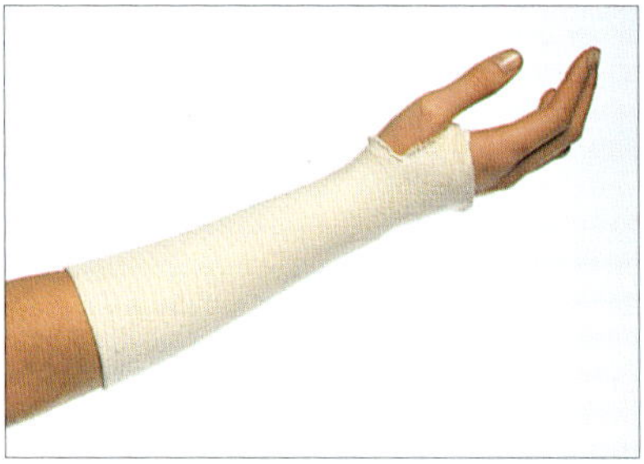

1 Cut a piece of gauze about 3 times the length of the limb you wish to bandage.

2 If there is an applicator, slide on the entire length of bandage and then very carefully slide the applicator over the injured limb.

3 Gently hold or tape the end of the bandage furthest from the top of the applicator and then pull the applicator away until there is a single layer of gauze over the limb.

4 Twist the applicator 2 or 3 times and then slide it over the limb once again.

5 Remove the applicator and secure the bandage, if necessary. Check that the bandage has not impeded circulation.

# SLINGS

A sling is normally made from a triangular bandage (*see page 140*), but it is certainly possible to improvise if one is not available.

## *Improvised Slings*

- The best way is to pin the sleeve of the injured arm to the shirt or coat near the shoulder area.
- If you don't have a pin, try using a tie or a pair of tights to twist around the arm and hook it round the neck (taking care not to tighten at the neck). This method provides less support but is useful for elevation.
- Tuck the hand of the injured limb into a buttoned shirt or jacket, at upper chest height.
- Fold up the bottom of a shirt or jumper, cradling the hand, forearm and elbow in the fold. Secure the edge of the garment to the opposite shoulder with a safety pin.

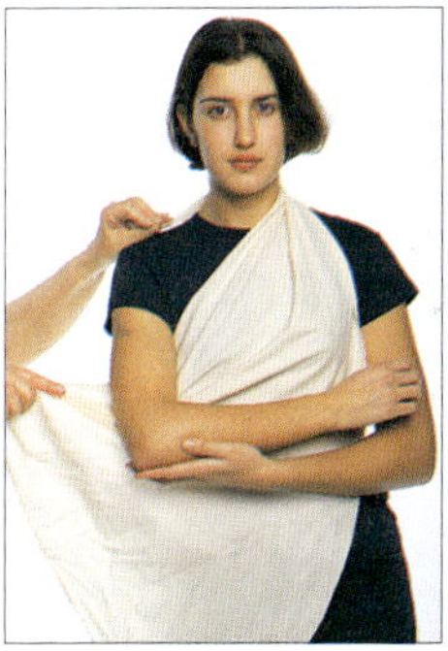

## *Arm Slings*

Arm slings support injured arms and wrists, and take the weight off an injured shoulder or collarbone.

1 Support the injured arm and gently ease the bandage between the arm and the chest. One point from the long end of bandage should run over the shoulder and around the neck.

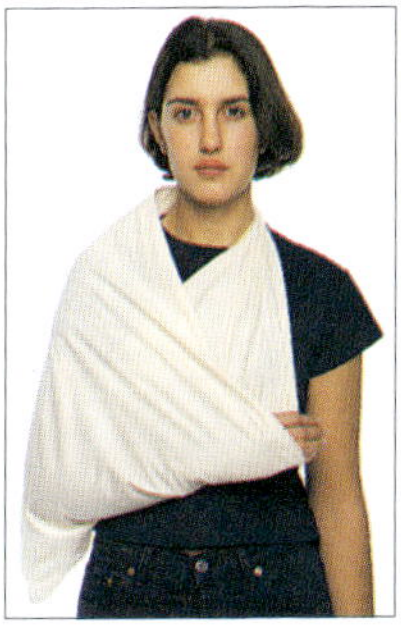

2 Lift the other point from the long end of the bandage up over the forearm to meet the other end at the shoulder.

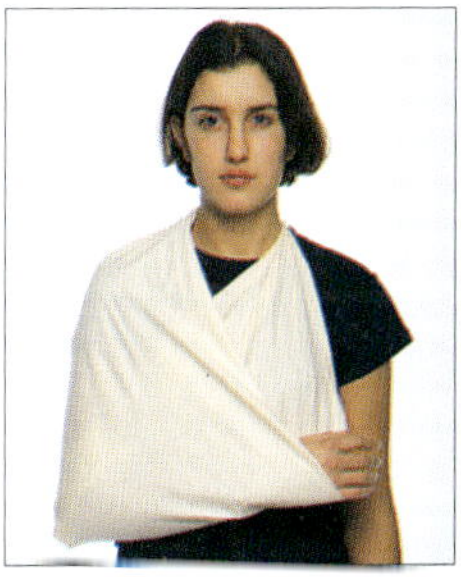

3 Tie a reef knot (*see page 147*) just below the level of the shoulder.

4 Pin the fabric at the end of the elbow to the bandage.

## *Elevation Slings*

An elevation sling is used when there are shoulder or chest injuries, or when the hand is bleeding.

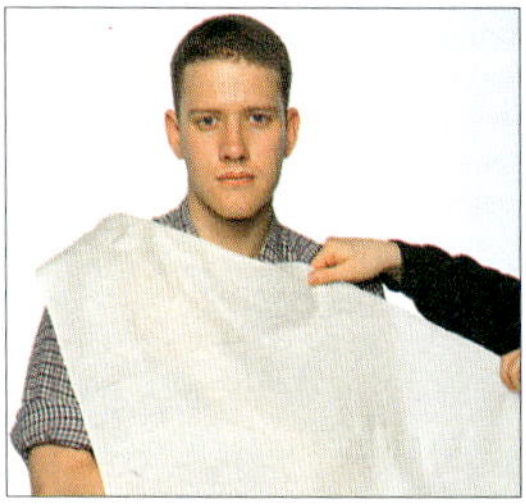

1 The arm on the injured side should be raised across the chest diagonally until the fingers rest on the opposite shoulder.

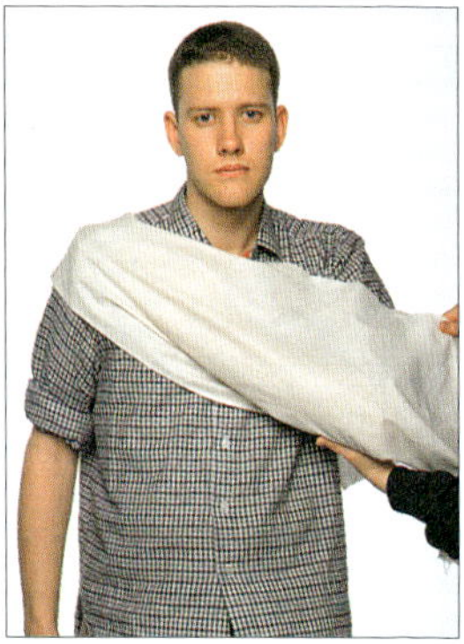

2 Lay an open triangular bandage over the forearm so that one end covers the hand and extends a few centimetres past the end of the fingers. The point will be across the elbow with plenty of room.

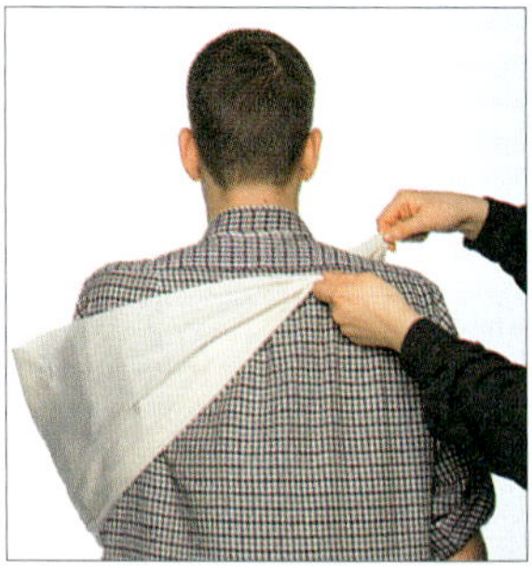

3 Gently lower the casualty's arm and, holding it carefully, tuck the base of the triangular bandage under the forearm and behind the elbow.

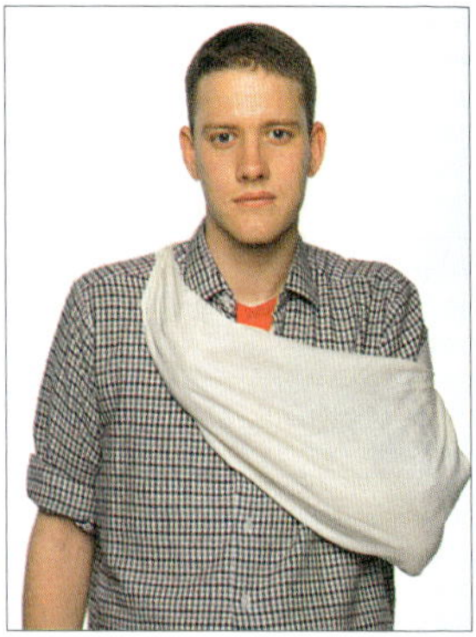

4 The end beneath the elbow should be brought up the back and across diagonally to meet the other end at the shoulder. Tie a reef knot (*see page 147*).

5 Tuck the ends of the bandage under the knot and fold the point forward so that all the edges of the bandage are underneath.

6 Fasten the bandage with a safety pin. Check that the circulation is not impeded.

> In an elevation sling the arm should be in a raised position, as high as possible within the bandage.

## *Tying a Reef Knot*

Reef knots are used to tie almost all bandages that are not taped or secured by a clip or pin (coloured cord has been used here for clarity).

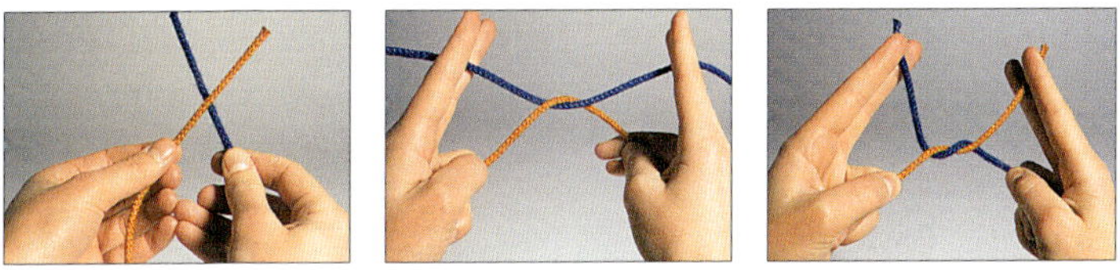

1 With one end of the bandage in each hand, take the left end over and then under the right.

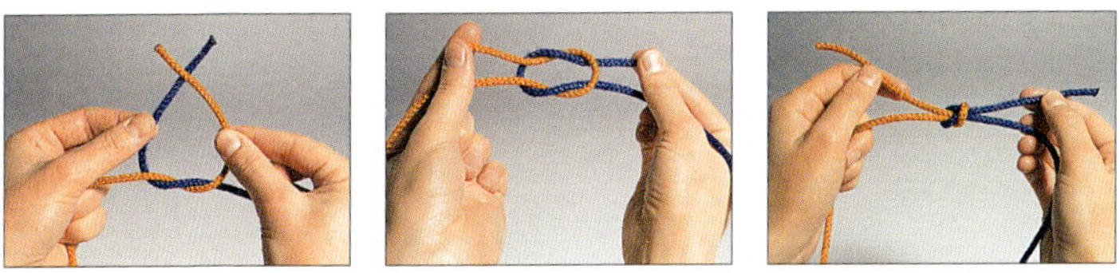

2 Take what is now the right end over and under the left and pull the knot tight.

3 To undo, simply pull the ends of the knot in opposite directions, then hold the knot and pull one end.

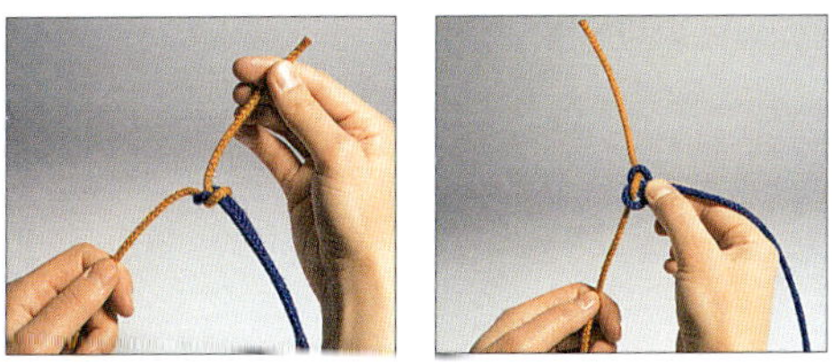

# SPLINTS

A splint is used to immobilise a limb and is used in cases of suspected fracture or when movement would make a condition such as profuse bleeding worse. Some First Aid kits carry small splints, and it is usually easy to improvise with a piece of board, or something firm that will prevent further movement.

In general, it is best to pad an injury with a rolled-up towel or with bandages, and then tie the injured limb to the body. An injured leg, for example, should be fixed to the uninjured leg.

Splint a limb if help will be more than 15–20 minutes coming and movement is not excessively painful.

## *Splinting a Leg*

1 Pad the thighs, knees and ankles of the injured leg with bandages, rolled-up towels or sheets. Gently bring the uninjured leg into line beside the injured limb.

2 Take a narrow bandage (*see page 140*) and tie a figure-of-eight bandage (*see page 141*) around the ankles and feet to immobilise the leg.

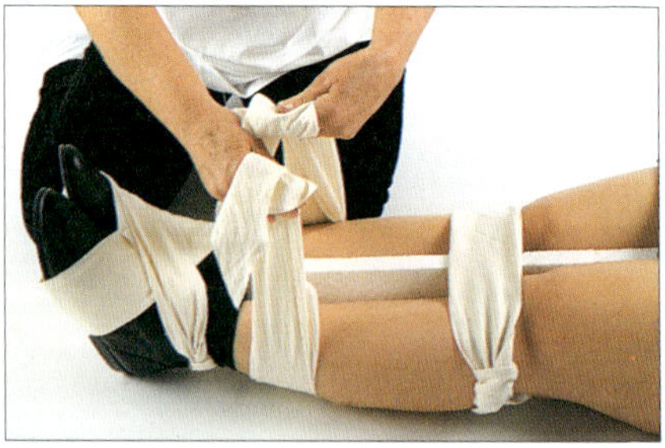

3 Take a broad bandage (*see page 140*) and tie around the legs above the knee and above the point of injury using a reef knot (*see page 147*).

Immobilise the legs in this manner for a broken pelvis or any suspected fractures or other injuries of the legs.

# LIFTING AND CARRYING

Moving a casualty is potentially dangerous and should never be done unless absolutely essential. It is necessary to move a casualty:

- When help is unavailable.
- When there is immediate danger to life.

If you must move a casualty, take steps to assess his injuries first so that anything which needs special support gets it. Always try to move a casualty in exactly the position in which he was found.

- NEVER move a casualty on your own if there is help available.
- NEVER move a casualty if your own safety or his life is endangered.
- NEVER assume that the casualty can support himself in a sitting or standing position.
- If you can, move the casualty in exactly the same position in which you found him.
- DO NOT move someone with severe crush injuries unless vital to their ongoing safety.
- DO NOT try to lift someone too heavy for you.
- DO NOT try to prevent a fall if you lose your balance or grip on the casualty – let him slide gently to the ground to avoid further injury.

GENERAL RULES FOR LIFTING

- Keep your feet apart and stand firmly over your centre of gravity.
- Lower yourself to the level of the casualty, bending your knees and not your back.
- Keeping your back straight, grip the casualty with your whole hands, keeping their weight as close to you as possible.
- Lift with your legs, not your back muscles, and use your shoulders to support the weight of the casualty.

## *One First-aider*

### DRAGGING

This should only be used if there is no way to lift the casualty and he cannot move on his own.

#### Holding the casualty by strong clothing

1 Cross the casualty's arms across the chest and support the head with a towel or article of clothing.

2 Grasp the casualty by the shoulders of his jacket, holding the head support in place as you do so.

3 Then drag the casualty by his clothing to a safe position.

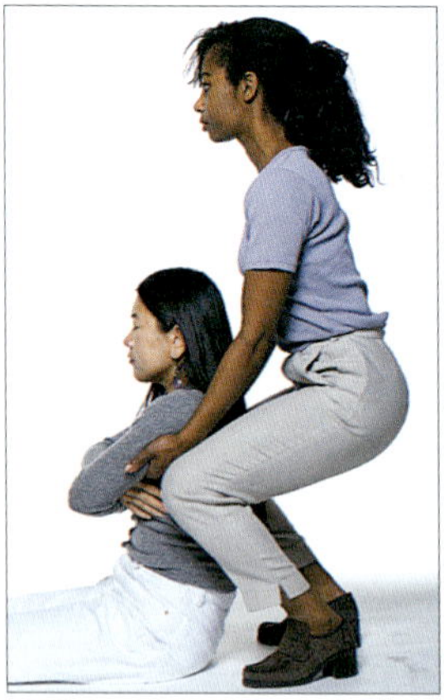

#### Holding the casualty bodily

1 If the casualty does not have a jacket or shirt, place your hands under her armpits and, using your forearms to support the head, drag the casualty to safety.

### THE HUMAN CRUTCH

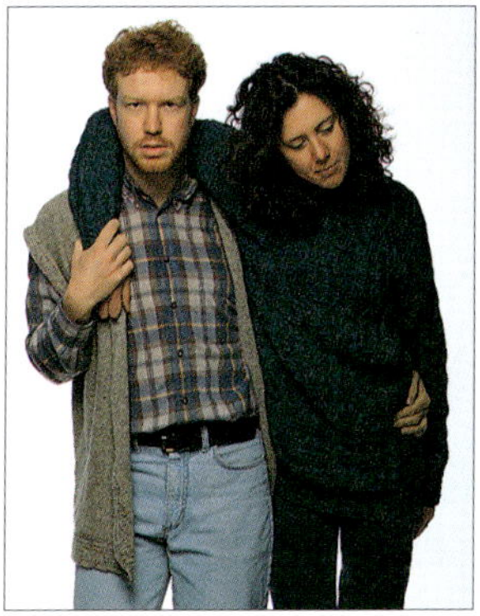

If the casualty is able to walk with assistance, this form of movement is best. The human crutch is not suitable if there has been an injury to the arm.

1 Place the casualty's arm around your neck, ensuring that you are on the uninjured side of the body.

2 Hold the hand of the arm around your neck and put your other arm around the casualty's waist, taking hold of the clothing at that point.

> **CHILDREN**
> Children should be cradled with the first-aider's hands under the knees and around the back and under the arms. A baby will need her head supported by the first-aider's arm.

There are a number of other lifts, including a fireman's lift, but these are best left to experienced first-aiders.

## *Two First-aiders*

Where there are two or more first-aiders it is possible to move single and multiple casualties with a minimum of disruption.

### THE FOUR-HANDED SEAT

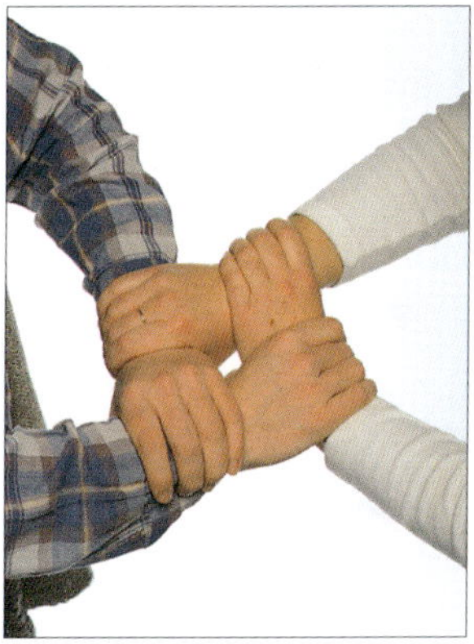

This carrying technique is used when the casualty is able to support himself with one or both arms.

1 Two first-aiders should face one another: one grasps his own right wrist with his left hand, and the other his left wrist with his right hand. Each then grasps the other's free wrist with their free hand.

2 Squat together, taking care to bend at the knees not the waist, and use your joined hands as a seat for the casualty

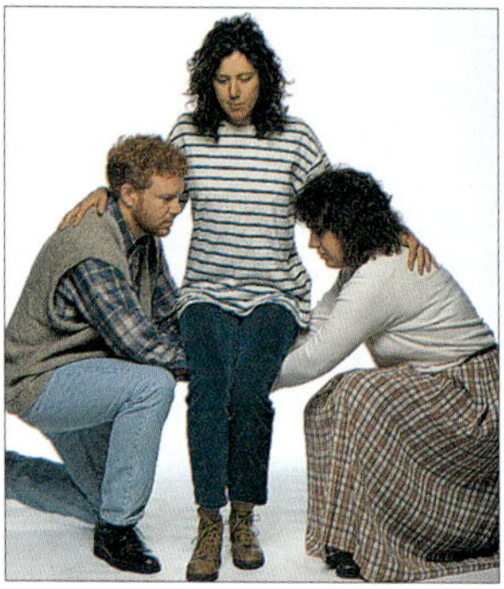

3 Let the casualty sit on your hands, placing her arms around your necks.

4 Rise together and synchronise your steps so that the casualty is not unduly jolted.

**THE TWO-HANDED SEAT**

This technique is used when the casualty is not able to support herself with one or both arms.

1 Two first-aiders should face one another on either side of the casualty and pass their forearms nearest to the casualty's body behind the casualty's back, just below the shoulder line.

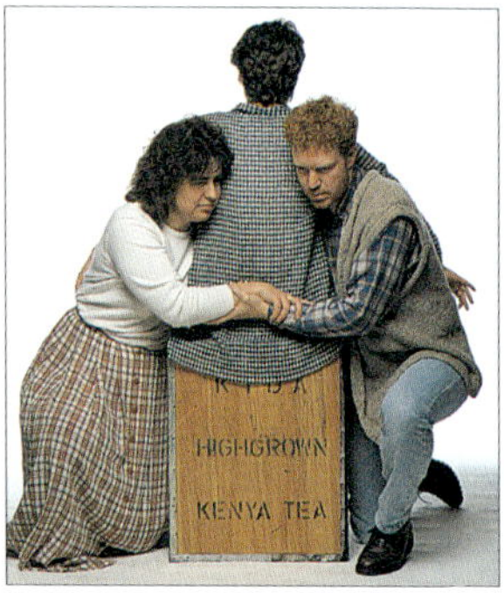


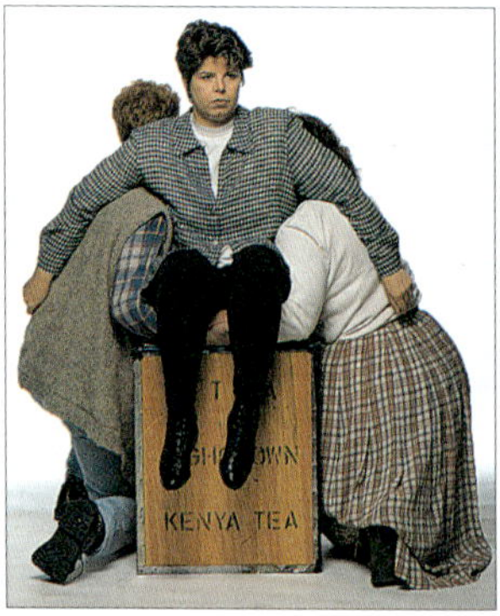


2 Grasp the casualty's clothing and raise the back slightly, passing the other arms under the middle of the casualty's thighs in order to grasp each other's wrists.

3 Supporting the casualty on your shoulders, rise together and synchronise your steps so that the casualty is not unduly jolted.

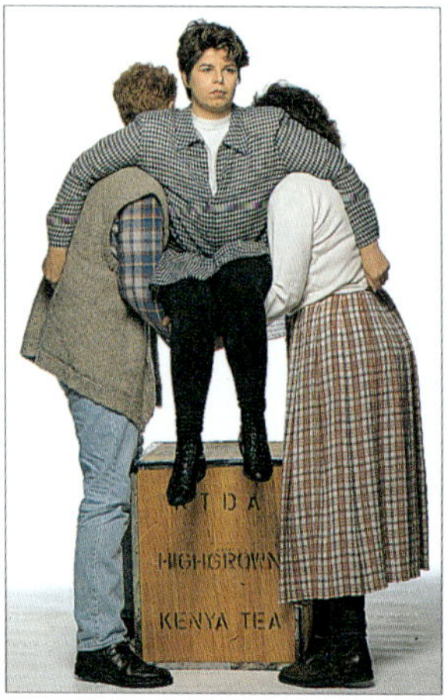

### CHAIRS

When there are stairs to contend with, or when you will have to walk a distance with the casualty, the chair method is most appropriate.

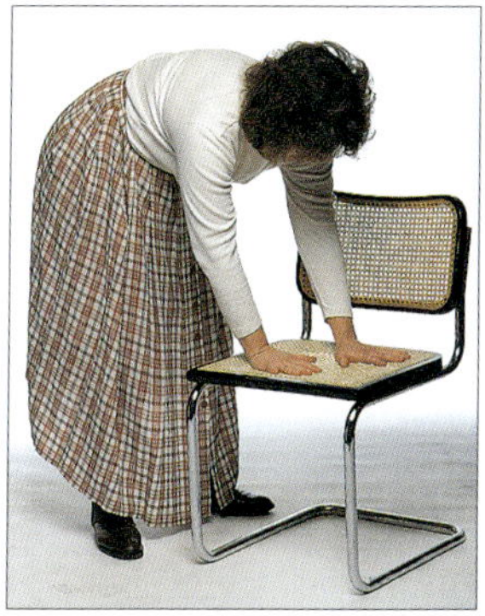

1 Check that the chair can support the casualty by putting your full weight on it, then seat the casualty so that she is comfortable.

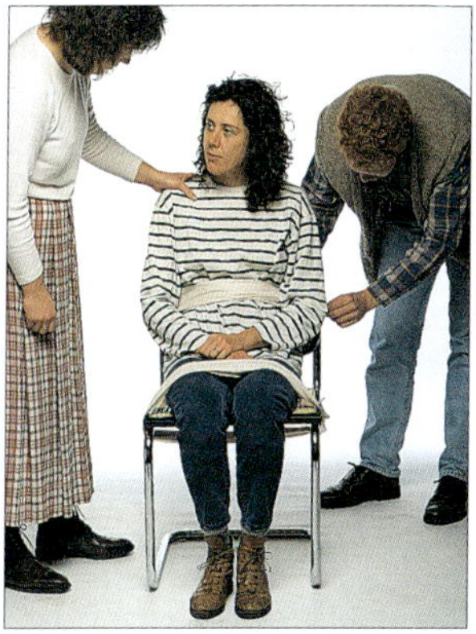

2 Secure her thighs and torso to the chair using belts, scarves or, if available, broad bandages (*see page 140*). Do not fasten them too tightly.

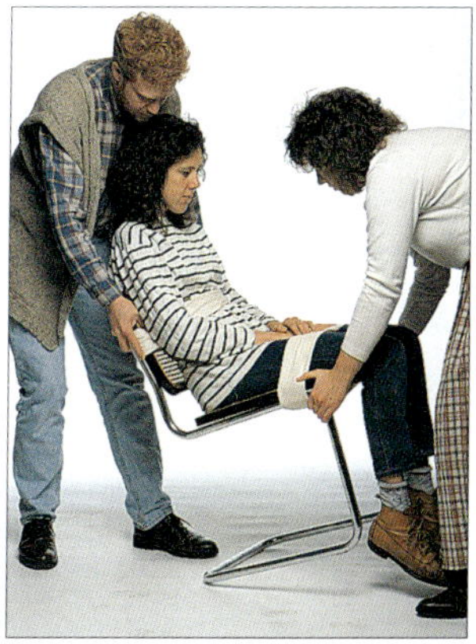

3 With one first-aider standing in front of the chair and another standing behind, tilt back the chair until it is at about a 30° angle.

4 To carry the chair, one first-aider stands in front of the casualty and the other behind. The first-aider in front can either face the casualty and walk backwards or have her back to the casualty and face forwards. The first-aider at the back of the casualty faces and moves forwards.

AVOID all unnecessary movement.

NEVER transport an unconscious casualty by chair.

Always reassure the casualty and tell her what you are doing.

# Stretchers with two or more first-aiders

NEVER move a casualty with a suspected neck or spine injury. Always immobilise any suspected fractures elsewhere in the body before moving.

Stretchers are necessary when the casualty must be transported over a long distance, or when a casualty is unable to walk and needs to be moved to shelter or to help. It is always best to wait for emergency medical attention whenever possible, as the team will always have specially designed stretchers that adapt to the requirements of the casualty.

If you do find you need a stretcher, you can improvise with a blanket, or by pushing the poles from two brooms or mops through the sleeves of two sturdy closed jackets with the arms tucked inside, one jacket forming the top half of the stretcher and the other the bottom.

A casualty should always be transported feet first except when she is being carried downstairs. The exception to this is a casualty suffering a stroke or any injury to the head and neck, under which circumstances she should be carried feet first downstairs.

## IMPROVISED STRETCHER

You will need four first-aiders for this procedure.

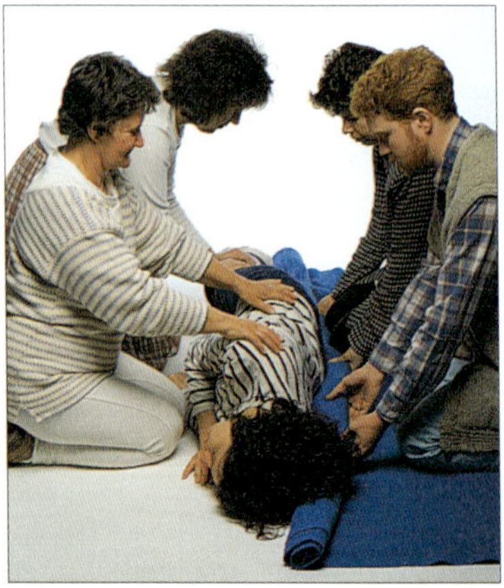

1 Roll a blanket until it is about half its width and roll the casualty on to her side so that the roll presses against her back. Always roll the casualty on her uninjured side.

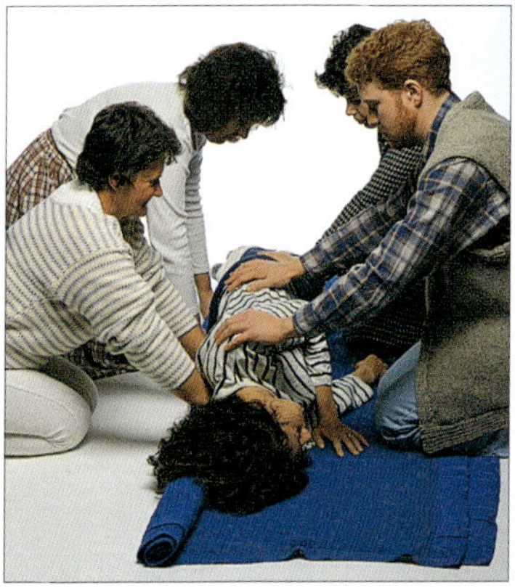

2 Ease the casualty back onto the blanket over the roll and on to her other side, facing away from the roll. Turn her only slightly if there is an injury present on that side.

3 Unroll the blanket slightly so that the casualty can lie flat.

4 Roll the other side of the blanket up till it touches the casualty.

5 Using the rolls as support for the casualty, the first-aiders should squat down together, taking care to bend from the knees not the back. Each first-aider should grasp the corner of the roll closest to them with one hand. With their other arms placed firmly beneath the casualty's body, they should rise together and synchronise their steps.

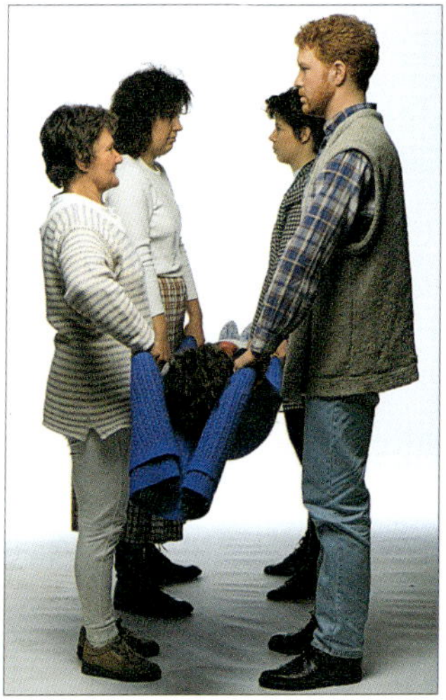

When it is necessary to transport a casualty by stretcher, let the most experienced first-aider co-ordinate the movements of the others and allow him to synchronise your steps.

# REMOVING CLOTHING

Only remove clothing if it is necessary to assess the extent of injury or to perform emergency treatment. Occasionally you may need to remove clothing which is constrictive, or if the casualty is overheated. In general, however, try to disturb the casualty as little as possible and always ask a conscious victim for permission before removing anything.

NEVER remove items of clothing unnecessarily since unintentional further harm can be caused to the casualty.

## REMOVING COATS, JACKETS OR SHIRTS

1 Seat the casualty, if possible, and pull off the coat from the shoulders.

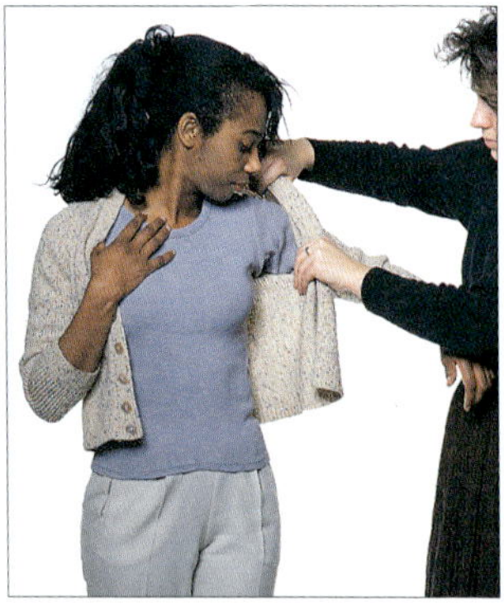

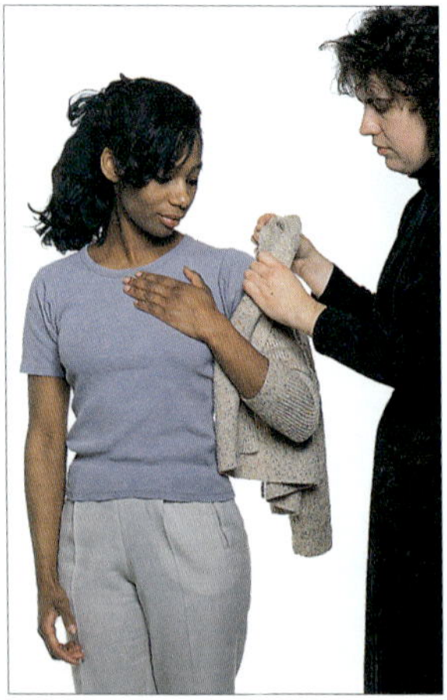

2 Bend the arm on the uninjured side and remove the coat from that side.

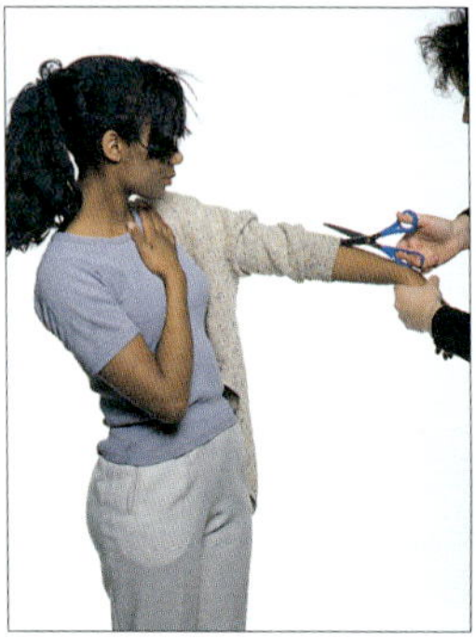

3 Slip the coat gently over the injured arm.

If you have trouble removing the coat, slit it on the side seam to make removal easier.

## REMOVING TROUSERS

1 Wherever possible, lift the trouser leg to reveal the injured part.

2 When complete removal is necessary, pull them down from the waist or cut up the leg of the trousers.

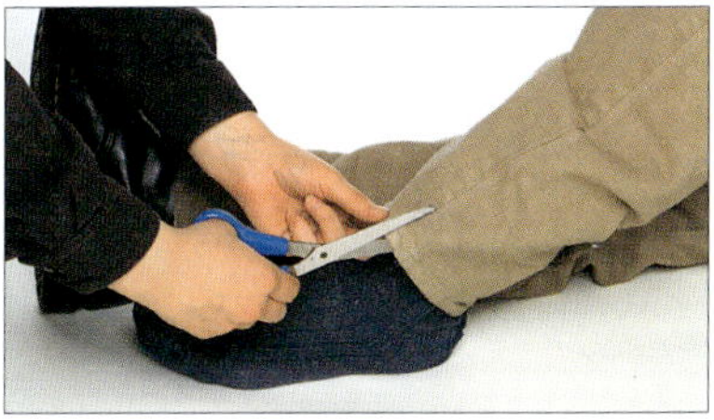

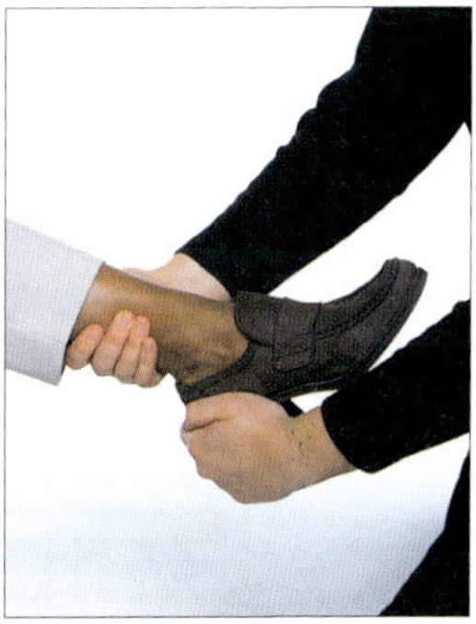

## REMOVING SHOES

1 Support the ankle and cut or undo any shoelaces.

2 Remove the shoe carefully.

If you have trouble removing shoes or boots, they can be cut up the back with a knife. Take care not to cause further injury.

## REMOVING SOCKS

1 If socks cannot be removed easily, insert two fingers into the top of the sock between the fabric and the front of the casualty's leg.

2 With a pair of scissors, carefully cut away the sock between your fingers, working your way to the toe, or until the sock can be slid off.

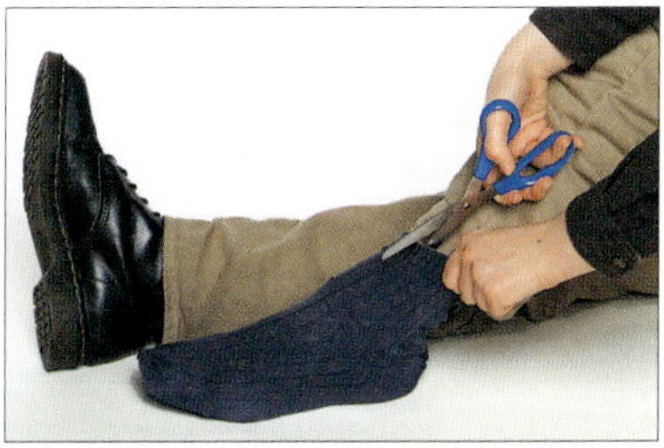

## REMOVING HELMETS

NEVER remove a helmet unless it is absolutely necessary – i.e. if the helmet is obstructing the airway or breathing, or if it is necessary to resuscitate (*see page 21*).

Always support the head and neck throughout the removal procedure.

Always ask the casualty to remove his own helmet, if possible.

Modern helmets are designed to protect the skull and face. Any movement caused by their removal may cause further damage. There are two main types of protective helmet:

**Open-face protective helmet**

1 Remove any sunglasses, goggles or eyeglasses before attempting to remove the helmet.

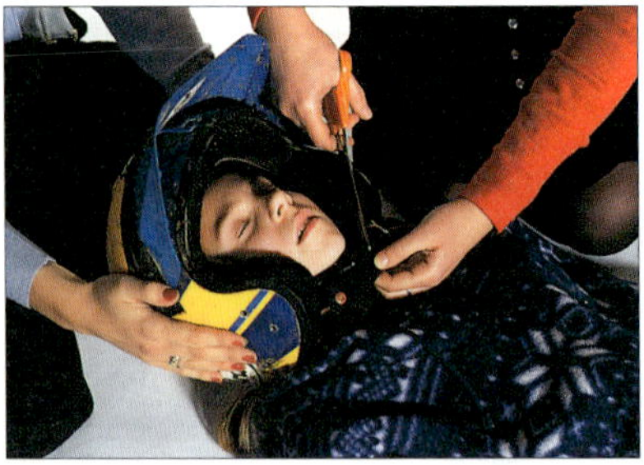

2 Unfasten or cut the strap under the chin.

3 There must be another first aider to hold the head and neck carefully while you force apart the helmet in order to lift it off.

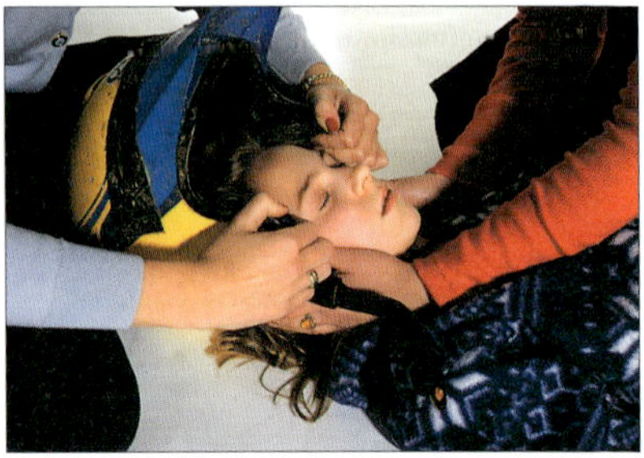

4 Remove the helmet with a smooth upwards and backwards movement and make sure the head is released gently.

**Full-face crash helmet**

These helmets should not be removed unless the casualty cannot breathe, is vomiting or has no circulation.

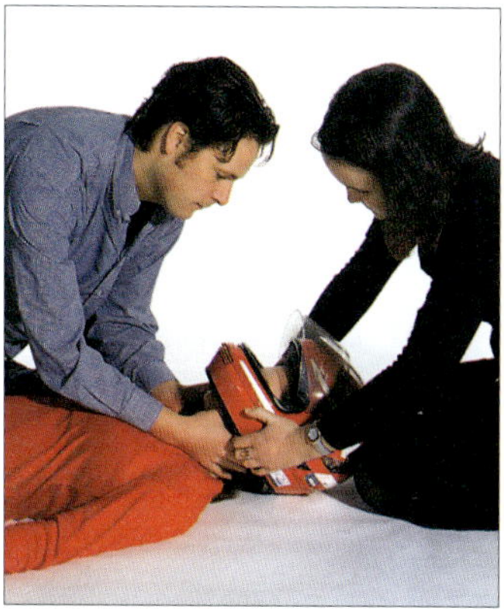

1 One first-aider holds the head firmly, preferably at the jaw.

2 The second first-aider undoes or cuts the chin strap so that the first first-aider can place his hands on each side of the head, inside the helmet.

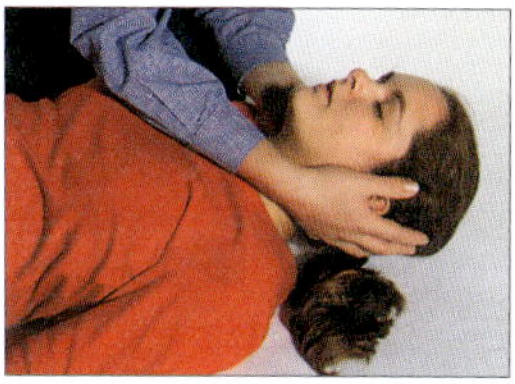

The first-aider supporting the head should aim to have his hands in this position, *inside the helmet*.

3 Ensuring that the casualty's head is well supported, the second first-aider tilts the helmet back so that the nose and chin are clear. Try to pull the helmet apart at the side.

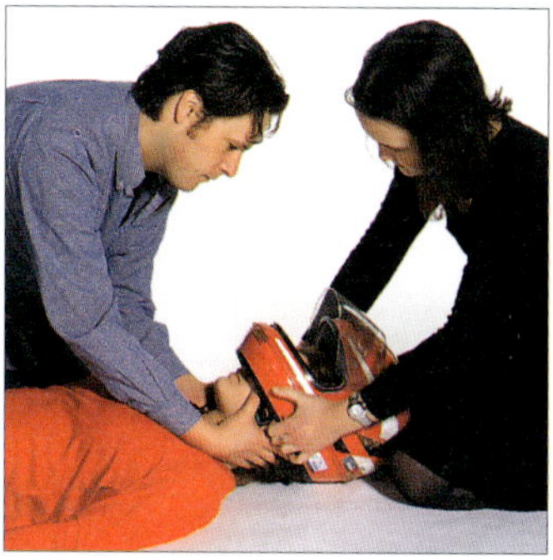

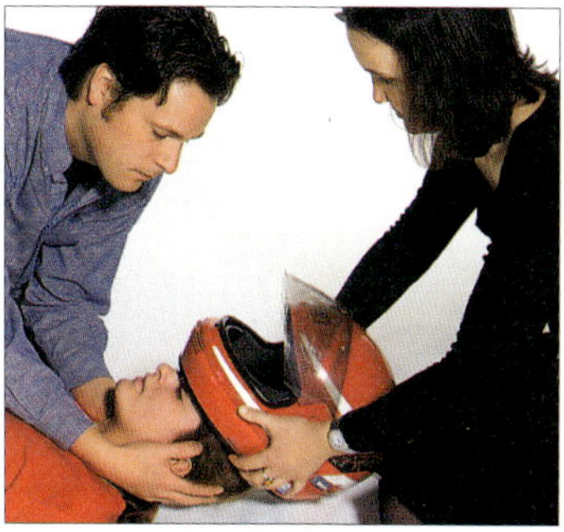

4 Tilt the helmet forward to move up and over the base of the skull, and lift it gently from the casualty. Do not move the head or neck unnecessarily.

# YOUR HOME FIRST AID KIT

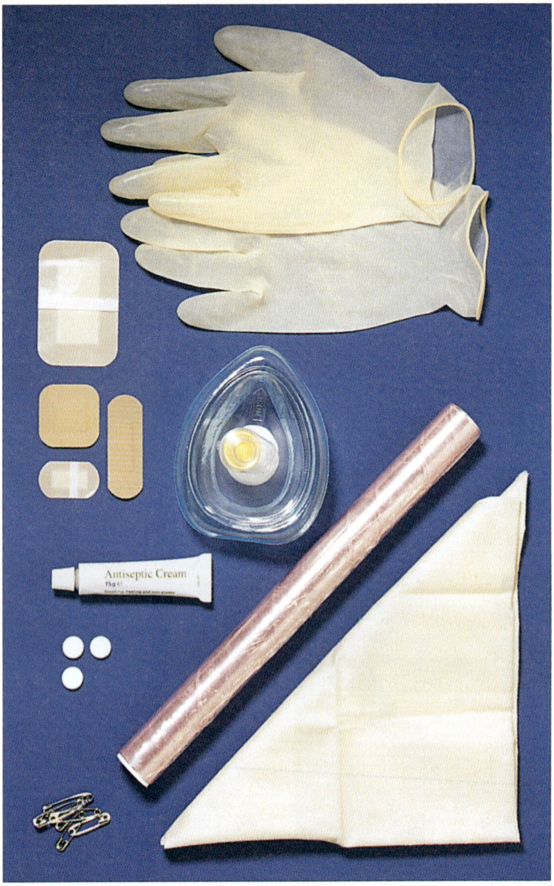

A First Aid kit is an invaluable piece of equipment for every household, car and workplace, and can be purchased at most chemists. If you decide to make your own, there are a few tips you should bear in mind:

- Use secure, airtight containers that will keep the contents clean and dry and make it portable.
- Keep your First Aid kit in an easily accessible position.
- Keep your First Aid kit out of reach of children.
- Keep it well stocked and check every few months to ensure that any medicines are not out of date.

# A BASIC KIT

- Simple instruction leaflet
- 2 pairs disposable gloves
- Face shield
- 12 plasters (adhesive dressings – at least one large)
- 2 triangular bandages
- 6 adult Paracetamol tablets
- Clingfilm/burns sheet for burns
- 6 safety pins
- Antiseptic

# AN INTERMEDIATE KIT

In addition to the contents of a Basic First Aid Kit (*see pages 160–61*), an Intermediate kit would include:

- Instruction leaflet
- 2 extra large dressings (also known as ambulance dressings)
- Elasticated self-adhesive bandage
- 4 additional triangular bandages
- 300ml (minimum) normal saline
- Sterile gauze
- Container powder for spillage of body fluids
- Scissors
- Record book, notepad, pens, labels*
- (A blanket and torch are desirable, separate from the kit)

Note: *These elements are used to record when items in the kit are used (record book), details about the casualty (notepad) and the precise action taken by a first-aider (labels, attached to the casualty).

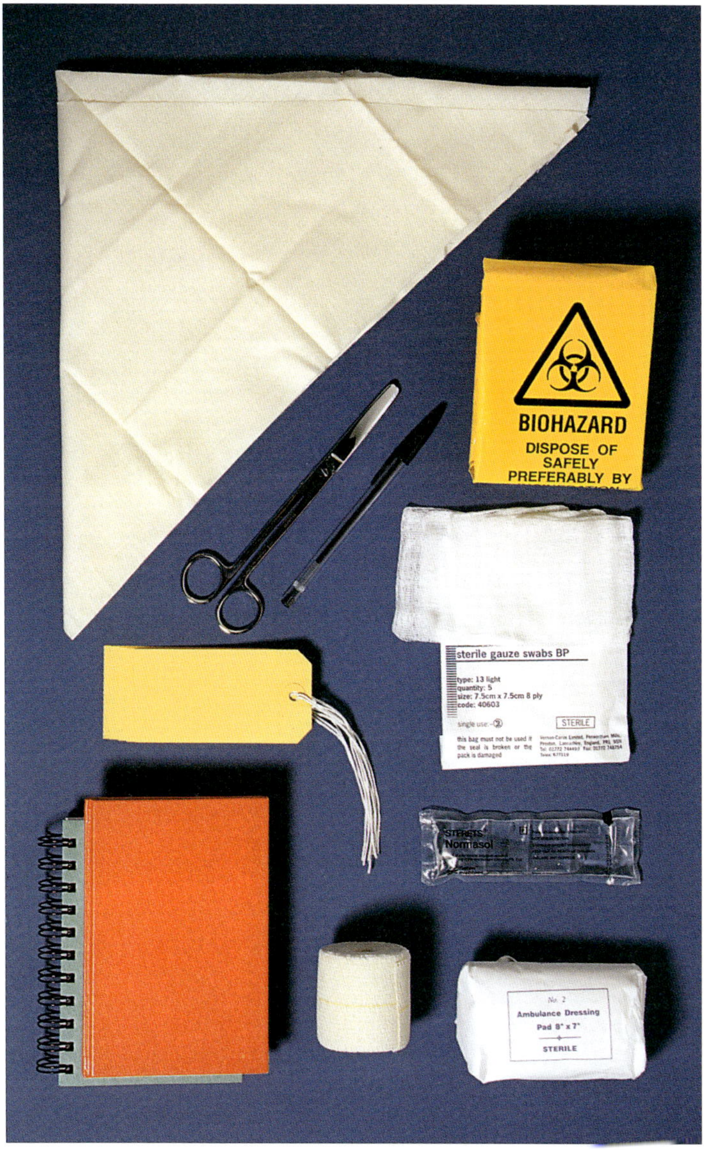
BIOHAZARD
DISPOSE OF
SAFELY
PREFERABLY BY
sterile gauze swabs BP
type: 13 light
quantity: 5
size: 7.5cm x 7.5cm 8 ply
code: 40603
single use
STERILE
this bag must not be used if the seal is broken or the pack is damaged
Normasol
No. 2
Ambulance Dressing
Pad 8" x 7"
STERILE

# FIRST AID KIT FOR THE CAR

In addition to the Basic First Aid Kit (*see pages 160–61*), you will need:

- Torch
- Blanket
- Hazard warning triangle
- Chocolate
- Snow shovel
- Tow-rope
- Whistle
- Polythene survival bag
- Extra triangular bandages
- Splint material
- Water flask
- Sleeveless jacket with reflective strips

# FIRST AID KIT FOR THE TRAVELLER

When going away, the contents of a first aid kit will vary according to where you are going, the condition of the areas in which you are travelling at the time and the time of year. In addition to the Basic First Aid Kit (*see pages 160–61*), you may need:

- Sterile travel pack
- Antibiotic ointment
- Anti-diarrhoea tablets
- Anti-nausea tablets
- Travel sickness tablets
- Oral rehydration salts
- Calamine lotion
- Sunscreen
- Insect repellent
- Vaccinations, if necessary
- Anti-malaria tablets, if necessary

Discuss your needs with your doctor or local pharmacist. Find out if you need vaccinations or anti-malaria tablets.

# FIRST AID FOR...

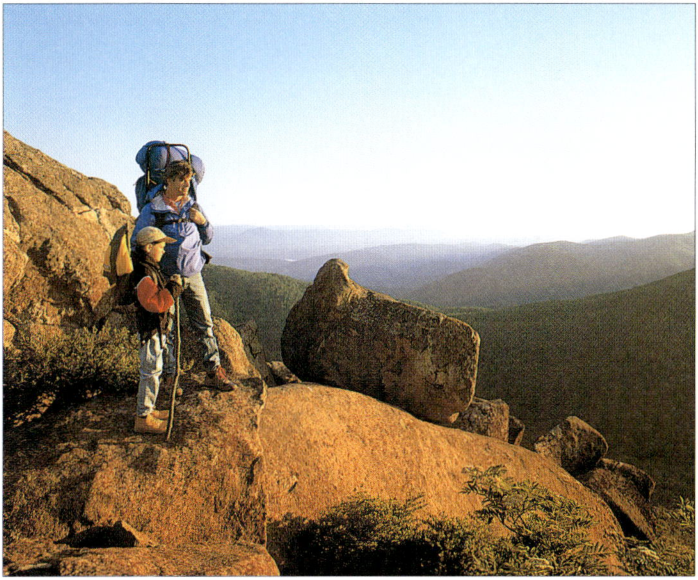

# ...BABIES AND CHILDREN

## An Emergency Checklist

The following is a quick-reference guide to some of the most common emergency situations and conditions involving children.

Allergic attack (*see page 54*)
Amputation (*see page 56*)
Asthma (*see page 57*)
Bleeding and wounds (*see pages 43, 58*)
Bruising (*see page 60*)
Burns (*see page 49, 62*)
Burns to the mouth and throat (*see page 51*)
Choking (*see page 68*)
Convulsions (*see page 72*)
Crush injuries (*see page 75*)
Cuts and grazes (*see page 58*)
Diarrhoea (*see page 117*)
Dislocations (*see page 118*)
Drowning (*see page 78*)
Electrical injuries (*see pages 65, 80*)
Eye injuries (*see page 120*)
Fainting (*see page 121*)
Fever (*see page 127*)
Foreign bodies: ear, eye, nose (*see pages 119, 120, 122*)
Fractured bones (*see page 81*)
Frostbite (*see page 90*)
Head injuries (*see page 94*)
Hiccups (*see page 170*)
Hypothermia (*see page 90*)
Joint and muscle injuries (*see pages 118, 125*)
Neck injuries (*see page 94*)
Poisoning (*see page 103*)
Shock (*see page 46*)
Strangulation (*see page 110*)
Travel sickness (*see page 130*)
Unconsciousness (*see page 36*)
Vomiting (*see page 117*)

Remember not to panic. Children are sensitive and they will respond adversely to anxiety.

For childhood illnesses *see pages 170–73*.

By their nature, children are prone to accidents and mishaps. The likelihood of an emergency situation arising is greater than for any other age group and above all it is important for parents and carers to be prepared to deal with these emergencies. Many emergency situations are handled differently for children, and throughout the book these differences appear in tinted boxes. Never assume a child should be treated as an adult. Children are not always able to describe their symptoms and it is all the more important to be familiar with the features of a condition or situation so that you can act swiftly.

## *What to Do in an Emergency*

There are 6 steps which you should remember in any emergency. Above all, stay calm.

1. **Assess the safety aspect.** Do so quickly. Think of:
- Will you or anyone else be injured by treating the child?
- Can you remove the source of danger from the child easily and safely?
- Should you move the child – bearing in mind that you should not move a casualty unless absolutely necessary.

2. **Assess the situation.** Do so quickly. Think of:
- The nature of the accident and how it happened.
- Who is injured and how badly.
- Is there any existing or continuing danger or is the child causing danger to anyone else?
- Should a doctor or ambulance be called?
- Do I need help?

3. **Follow the ABC of resuscitation** (*see page 21*) and be prepared to resuscitate (*see page 28*).

4. ☎ **Ring for help.** Call for an ambulance or doctor.

5. **Address injuries.** Deal with:
- Unconsciousness.
- Bleeding.
- Shock.
- Burns.
- Any other injuries.

6. **Stay with the child. Provide constant reassurance.** If she is seriously injured, check breathing and circulation (*see page 23*) constantly.

## *Safety Points for Babies and Children*

- Watch out for strange or over-zealous dogs both at home and out of doors.
- Don't leave a dog and a child alone together.
- Keep knives, scissors, screwdrivers and all sharp tools out of reach.
- Keep sewing materials out of reach.
- Replace plate-glass windows and French doors with safety glass.
- Keep electrically powered appliances out of reach.
- Never leave a baby or toddler alone in a room.
- Furniture which is not solid or steady should be replaced or put to one side until the child is older.
- Beware of swing doors and those with automatic closures.
- Use a flex-free kettle and keep it well out of the reach of children.
- All fires need guards.
- Avoid paraffin heaters if you can.
- Watch the hob – make sure all saucepan handles are turned inwards. Even the outside of an oven can be very hot and cause serious burns.
- Check the hot water temperature. If it runs too high, radiators and taps can lead to serious burns.
- Avoid using hot-water bottles for small children. Use only hand-hot water for older children.
- Never leave a baby or child alone with food or a bottle.
- Don't let a baby or child play with anything small enough to be swallowed.
- Don't give nuts to pre-school children.
- Don't give grapes or cherries to children unless they are cut up.
- Never leave a child alone in the bath.
- Help your child learn basic swimming skills and help her to feel confident in water but to be aware of the risks.
- Cover garden pools or water butts.
- Supervise paddling pools at all times.
- Empty paddling pools at the end of every session.
- Teach your child to avoid plugs and light switches.
- Don't give a child an electric blanket.
- Make sure all of your appliances are earthed.
- Avoid trailing flexes.
- Take care around balconies.
- Beware of rugs on polished floors.
- Use safety gates on the stairs, at the top and the bottom.
- Watch steps in the garden. Consider a safety fence.
- Buy a medicine cabinet with a safety lock. Do not keep medicines anywhere but in this cabinet.

- Don't allow your child to play with empty medicine containers.
- Be vigilant in other people's homes.
- Keep all cleaning substances in a locked or high cupboard.
- Lock garden sheds and garages.
- Teach your child how to cross the road safely, but do not allow him to do so on his own until the age of 8.
- Safety check all bicycles.
- Strongly recommend your child wears a safety helmet when he is riding a bicycle.
- Use approved carseats for babies and small children until the age of 7.
- Keep children away from plastic bags and empty trunks or boxes.
- Don't give a baby a pillow when she is sleeping.
- Use a high SPF (15 –25) sunscreen if your child is in the sun. Reapply regularly. Babies should not be exposed to sun at all.
- Put a wide-brimmed sunhat on children and avoid midday sun.
- Sterilise all baby's feeding equipment.
- Always use a safety harness in a high chair.
- Never leave your front door open.
- Buy toys that have an approved safety mark.
- Buy only non-toxic paints and writing materials.
- Make sure your baby's cot is deep enough to prevent him from climbing out.
- Always put your baby to sleep on her back or side, which is believed to reduce the risk of cot death.
- When your child begins to climb out of his cot, move him to a bed.
- Make sure your child cannot climb out of any windows in the house. Fit safety catches.

There are a number of childhood illnesses that commonly occur. They can all be distressing, to the child and his parents and carers.

NEVER exceed recommended doses – these are always specified on medications, and special medicines are available for babies and children.

Discuss immunisation for your child against measles, mumps, rubella and whooping cough with a doctor. First immunisations can take place when the baby is 8 weeks old.

## *Croup*

Croup is caused by an inflammation of the main airway to the lungs. It affects young children and causes a partial obstruction to the airway through the voice box. Hence, breathing is difficult and there is a harsh and painful cough. The characteristic bark is known as stridor. Croup is fairly common in small children, usually as a result of a viral infection that causes the lining of the larynx and trachea to swell. There may be blueness to the skin and an alarming pulse rate. Your child may be very restless and distressed. Very severe croup may close the airway, but is uncommon.

WHAT TO DO

1. Help your child to sit up in bed. Prop him up with pillows and provide constant reassurance. The condition is made worse by panic. In the case of a baby, put pillows under the mattress so that it rests at an angle.
2. Fill a room with steam. Use a kettle or a vaporiser in a sealed bedroom or run the hot water taps in the bathroom. Sit in the room until your child is calmer and finding breathing easier.
3. If there is no obvious improvement, call your doctor.

The disease is infectious.

Children may also develop a condition called epiglottitis that has many of the same symptoms as croup, but is accompanied by a very high fever. This is an emergency situation and medical assistance will be required immediately.

# Chickenpox

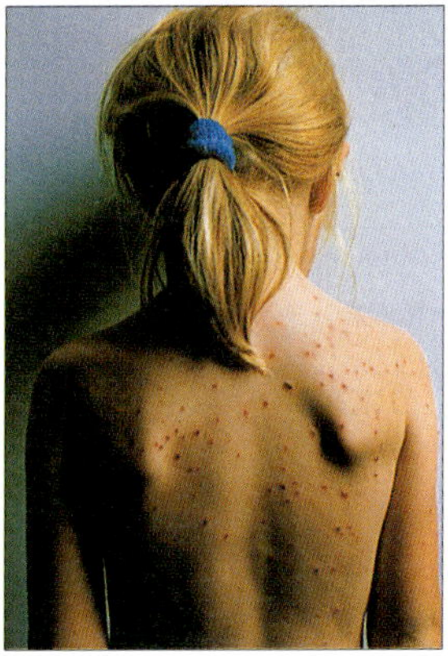

The symptom is a rash of small blisters, and the child may have a temperature. The rash starts on the chest and back before spreading to other areas of the body.

WHAT TO DO

1. If the child is very unwell or distressed, seek medical attention.
2. Give plenty to drink.
3. Give Paracetamol to bring down the temperature.
4. Reduce the itchiness by bathing the child and putting Calamine lotion on the rash. Make sure loose-fitting clothes are worn.

> The disease is infectious from the day before the rash appears, until the spots are dry.

# Measles

Symptoms are a feverish illness and a rash of slightly raised red spots which develop on the third or fourth day. The rash is not itchy but the child has a high temperature and a cough and will be ill for about a week.

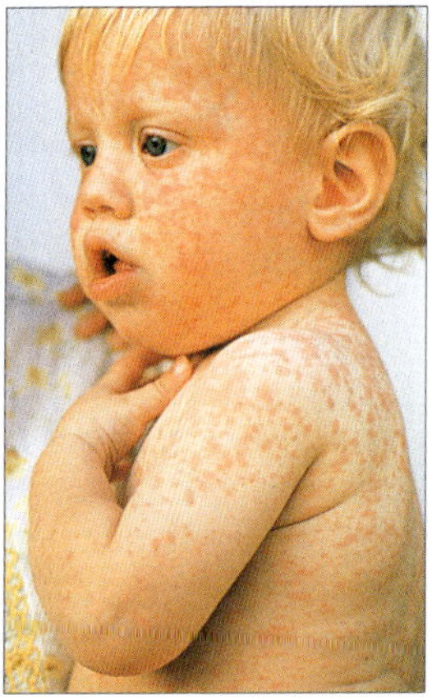

WHAT TO DO

1. Call for a doctor.
2. Make the child rest and give him plenty to drink – warm drinks will ease the cough.
3. Give Paracetamol to bring down the temperature.
4. Put Vaseline round the lips to protect the skin.
5. Wash the eyelids with warm water.

> The disease is infectious from a few days before the rash appears until five days after it goes.

## Mumps

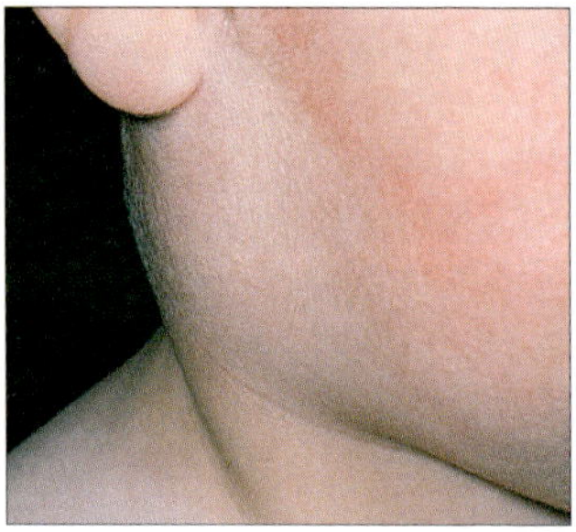

The first symptom may be pain round the ear or when chewing. Swelling will then develop under the jaw by the ear – this often starts at one ear and may then occur at the other.

WHAT TO DO

1. Give Paracetamol for the pain in the swollen glands.
2. Give plenty to drink.

Avoid giving fruit juice drinks. They make the saliva flow and this can be painful.

If the child has stomach-ache and is being sick, see a doctor.

The disease is infectious from a few days before the symptoms develop until the swelling goes down.

## Rubella (German Measles)

The child does not usually feel ill. Symptoms are a cold and a rash of flat spots which appears two days later. The rash begins on the face and then spreads. Glands in the back of the neck may swell.

WHAT TO DO

1. Give plenty to drink.

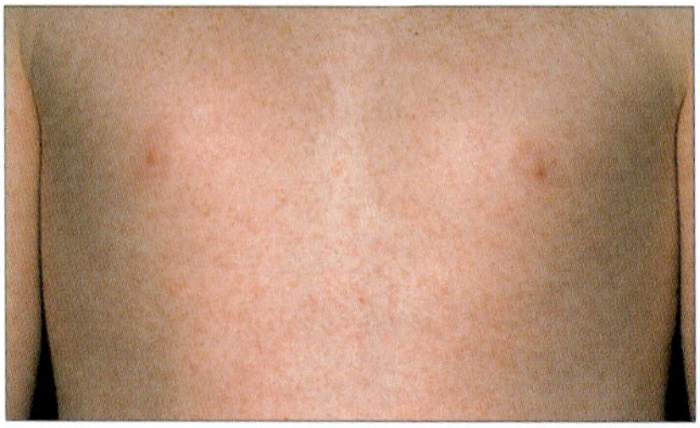

NEVER let your child come into contact with anyone who is pregnant or who is trying to become pregnant.

If your child came into contact with anyone who is pregnant before you know about the illness, let them know.

The disease is infectious from a few days before the illness starts until a week after the rash first appears.

## *Whooping cough*

The symptom is a cough which gets worse. Coughing bouts start after two weeks – these are very tiring and make breathing difficult. There may be a whooping noise when the child inhales after coughing. The coughing fits will not begin to calm down for a few weeks.

If the cough gets worse and the fits of coughing happen more often, see a doctor.

The disease is infectious from the first signs of illness until about six weeks after coughing first started.

## *Hiccups*

Many children suffer from hiccups which are normally harmless. Occasionally an attack can go on for several hours, causing worry, pain and distress. In those circumstances, seek medical advice.

# ...DRIVERS AND PASSENGERS

## *An Emergency Checklist*

The following is a quick-reference guide to some of the most common emergency situations and conditions associated with driving and road traffic accidents.

Amputation (*see page 56*)
Bleeding and wounds (*see pages 43, 58*)
Bruising (*see page 60*)
Burns (*see page 49, 62*)
Burns to the mouth and throat (*see page 51*)
Chemical burns (*see page 64*)
Crush injuries (*see page 75*)
Cuts and grazes (*see page 58*)
Dislocations (*see page 118*)
Electrical injuries (*see pages 65, 80*)
Fainting (*see page 121*)
Fire (*see pages 49, 108*)
Foreign bodies: ear, eye, nose (*see pages 119, 120, 122*)
Fractured bones (*see page 81*)
Head injuries (*see page 94*)
Impalement (*see page 100*)
Joint and muscle injuries (*see pages 118, 125*)
Neck injuries (*see page 94*)
Poisoning (*see page 103*)
Shock (*see page 46*)
Travel sickness (*see page 130*)

Road accidents can occur anywhere and you should be prepared to perform First Aid: to have a good First Aid kit on hand wherever you go.

(*See* **First Aid Kit for the Car**, *page 164*).

# ...THE WORKPLACE

## *An Emergency Checklist*

The following is a quick-reference guide to some of the most common emergency situations and conditions encountered in the workplace.



First aid in the workplace is governed by various regulations and legislation. Employers are required to do a risk assessment in all areas relating to health and safety. The health and safety of workers is, within reason, the responsibility of the employer. This responsibility is defined and controlled by the Health and Safety Executive.

Every company should be aware of the Approved Code of Practice and Guidance that was published in 1997 by the HSE. This outlines:

- Selection and training of first-aiders.
- Assessment of first-aid needs.
- The contents of a first aid kit.
- First-aider competencies.
- Record keeping of injuries and illness and the steps taken to administer treatment.

Accidents can happen anywhere, and your workplace First Aid Kit should contain items that prepare you for any eventuality. The kit must be accessible. You will be provided with a list of what is necessary: keep an extra supply of dressings, bandages, scissors, tweezers, gloves and eye solutions (particularly if you work with chemicals).

If you do administer first aid in the workplace, you must file a signed report with the following details:

- The date, time and place of the incident.
- The name and job of the injured or ill person.
- Details of the injury/illness and what first aid was given.
- What happened to the person immediately afterwards (for example, 'went home' / 'went back to work').
- Name and signature of the first-aider or person dealing with the incident.

## *Factory Work*

In a factory, there may be scope for more serious accidents such as crush injuries, impalement and amputation (*see pages 75, 100 and 56*).

## *Fire*

If you are confronted by fire, implement your workplace fire procedure. Then:

- ☎ Call for the emergency services. Provide as much information as you can.
- If there are chemicals that may give off poisonous or inflammable fumes, make the emergency services aware of them. Take urgent steps to seal fumes off, by closing doors, and then exit as quickly as you can.
- Make sure that all staff are evacuated without fuss.
- Do not enter a burning room or building.
- If you are trapped in a room in a burning building, shut and seal the door with towels or a coat at the base. Open a window and stay by it.

## *Electricity*

Electrical injuries may be more serious in the workplace because many businesses, in particular factories, have more powerful installations.

- Do not approach a casualty until you are certain that the power has been turned off.
- Do not go within 18 metres (60 feet) of the incident if the voltage is high and ring the emergency services, providing as much detail as you can about the accident.
- When the power is shut off, treat as for electrical injuries (*see page 80*).

# ...THE ELDERLY

## *An Emergency Checklist*

The following is a quick-reference guide to some of the most common emergency situations and conditions affecting the elderly.

Asthma (*see page 57*)
Bleeding and wounds (*see pages 43, 58*)
Breathing problems (*see pages 57, 66 and 112*)
Bruising (*see page 60*)
Burns and scalds (*see page 49, 62*)
Cardiac arrest (*see page 66*)
Choking (*see page 68*)
Cuts and grazes (*see page 58*)
Dehydration (*see page 117*)
Diabetes (*see page 77*)
Diarrhoea (*see page 117*)
Drowning (*see page 78*)
Epilepsy (*see page 72*)
Fainting (*see page 121*)
Fire (*see pages 49, 108, 179*)
Foreign bodies: ear, eye, nose (*see pages 119, 120, 122*)
Fractures (*see page 81*)
Frostbite (*see page 90*)
Head injuries (*see page 94*)
Heart attack (*see page 66*)
Hypoglycaemia (*see page 77*)
Hypothermia (*see page 90*)
Nausea and vomiting (*see page 117*)
Neck injuries (*see page 94*)
Poisoning (*see page 103*)
Stroke (*see page 112*)
Unconsciousness (*see page 36*)

Elderly people are more prone to illness and injury – partly because old age brings with it many health problems, but also because many elderly people live alone, often on a limited income. Some of the problems more common in old age include: diabetes, which brings with it the possibility of hypoglycaemia (*see page 77*) and coma; osteoporosis, which means that even a slight fall may cause a fracture (*see page 81*); atherosclerosis, a common cause of heart attack (*see page 66*); and stroke (*see page 112*).

Many elderly people suffer from impaired sight or hearing, which makes accidents more likely to happen.

The elderly are also more likely to suffer from dementia, the effects of which are exacerbated by poverty and poor housing conditions. There may be incontinence and also confusion, leading to a failure to eat and keep warm. Confusion in older people may also lead to carelessness with fires and electrical appliances. As with all age groups, it is essential that smoke alarms are fitted.

## *Fire*

### PREVENTING FIRE

Help the Aged suggests running through the following checklist before you go out, or retire for the night:

1. Have you turned off the burners and rings on your cooker?
2. Have you turned off the heaters and placed the guard in front of open fires?
3. Have you unplugged electrical appliances not in use?
4. Have you closed all the internal doors?
5. Have you unplugged your electric blanket if it is the type that should not be left on overnight?
6. Have you safely disposed of all smoking materials, including cigarette and pipe ash?

**What to do if there is a fire:**

- Close all internal doors.
- Make sure everyone leaves the house.
- ☎ Call for the emergency services.
- Provide the emergency services with your correct address.
- Wait outside until help arrives. Do not go back into the house for any reason.

**If you are trapped in a burning building:**

- Find a room that is not burning, if possible with a window.
- Close the door behind you and open the window.
- Block the foot of the door with towels, bedclothes or anything else.
- ☎ Attract the attention of a passer-by, or call for the emergency services yourself.

# Accidents in the Home

Failing vision, slower reflexes and muscle weakness make hazards easily avoided by younger people significant for the elderly and falls are common.

Because of these risks, every effort should be made to avoid hazards in the environment of the elderly such as loose mats on polished floors, damaged floor coverings, carelessly disposed electric cables, poorly lit stairs or corridors and icy paths. Help the Aged offers the following advice checklists:

- Make sure all corridors and stairs are well lit.
- Put handrails on both sides of stairs.
- Sturdy shoes with ridged, rubberised soles and non-slip heels will help to give you extra stability if unsteadiness is a problem.
- Don't lift heavy objects or bags of groceries. Try not to carry too much at once and try to get help with lifting heavy objects.
- Rearrange the furniture in your main living area to help you move around more freely and save you bumping into things.
- Make sure there are no trailing flexes or rucked-up carpets to trip you over.
- Bifocal glasses are unsettling to walk around in at first. Special care will be needed on the stairs.

## In the Kitchen

- Plan a clear space near the sink and cooker to put things down.
- Avoid straining to reach high shelves or bending into low cupboards. Place things you use every day where they are easy to get at.
- Use a tin opener that works easily to save injuring yourself.
- A timer will help to remind you that you have left something cooking.
- Spills on the floor should be cleaned up immediately to prevent you slipping on them.
- Gas appliances need to be serviced regularly by a registered installer.

## In the Bathroom

- Running the cold water before the hot, or running them together will mean the bath is never hot enough to scald you.
- A fitted carpet in the bathroom is safer than vinyl and loose mats.
- Raising your arms when leaning over the wash basin to shampoo your hair could cause you to feel faint. You could avoid this by asking someone to help you or by washing your hair in the bath.

- Always leave the bathroom door unlocked.
- If possible, arrange for someone else to be in the house when you take a bath.

## *In the Bedroom*

- Electric fires and heaters can easily set light to bedclothes, furniture and curtains unless they are kept well clear.
- Electric blankets don't last for ever – look for danger signs like frayed fabric, worn flex and scorch marks. Switch off electric underblankets before you get into bed.
- You can avoid feeling faint by taking your time and sitting on the edge of the bed for a minute or so before getting to your feet.
- Tripping is easy to do, so watch for a loose dressing gown tie or sheets on the floor.
- Can you switch on your bedroom lamp easily? A torch by the bed may also be helpful.

# ...OUTDOOR ACTIVITIES, PUBLIC EVENTS AND SPORT

## *An Emergency Checklist*

The following is a quick-reference guide to some of the most common emergency situations and conditions in crowds.

Allergic attack (*see page 54*)
Bites and stings (*see page 114*)
Bleeding and wounds (*see pages 43, 58*)
Breathing problems (*see pages 56, 66, 112*)
Cardiac arrest (*see page 66*)
Choking (*see page 68*)
Concussion (*see page 71*)
Crush injuries (*see page 75*)
Cuts and grazes (*see page 58*)
Dislocations (*see page 118*)
Drowning (*see page 78*)
Eye injuries (*see page 120*)
Fainting (*see page 121*)
Fire (*see pages 49, 108*)
Foreign bodies: ear, eye, nose (*see pages 119, 120, 122*)
Frostbite (*see page 90*)
Fractures (*see page 81*)
Head and neck injuries (*see page 94*)
Heart attack (*see page 66*)
Heat stroke (*see page 99*)
Hypothermia (*see page 90*)
Neck injuries (*see page 94*)
Nosebleed (*see page 122*)
Poisoning (alcohol) (*see page 103*)
Sprains and strains (*see page 125*)
Stroke (*see page 112*)
Sunburn (*see page 126*)
Toothache and knocked-out teeth (*see page 128*)

As a result of the Lord Justice Taylor inquiry into the Hillsborough Stadium Disaster Report, recommendations have now been adopted for minimum first aid standard at sports stadia and other places where large

numbers of people gather for recreational activity.
The minimum requirements laid out by the Taylor recommendations are:

- One trained first-aider per 1,000 spectators.
- One or more approved designated First Aid rooms.
- One trained medical practitioner at any event with more than 2,000 spectators.
- One ambulance authority-approved, fully equipped ambulance at any event with a crowd of 5,000.
- A Major Incident Equipment vehicle designed and equipped for up to 50 casualties deployed in addition to other ambulances in attendance when a crowd in excess of 25,000 is expected.

Sport and sports events are more likely to involve injury to muscle and bone than any other type of event, and steps must be taken to provide equipment to deal with them.

# ...TRAVELLERS

## *An Emergency Checklist*

The following is a quick-reference guide to some of the most common emergency situations and conditions encountered by travellers.

Allergic attack (*see page 54*)
Bites and stings (*see page 114*)
Bleeding and wounds (*see pages 43, 58*)
Cuts and grazes (*see page 58*)
Diarrhoea (*see page 117*)
Drowning (*see page 78*)
Fainting (*see page 121*)
Food poisoning (*see page 90*)
Foreign bodies: ear, eye, nose (*see pages 119, 120, 122*)
Frostbite (*see page 90*)
Heart attack (*see page 66*)
Heat exhaustion and heat stroke (*see page 98*)
Hypothermia (*see page 90*)
Nosebleed (*see page 122*)
Poisoning (*see page 103*)
Sprains and strains (*see page 125*)
Sunburn (*see page 126*)
Toothache and knocked-out teeth (*see page 128*)
Travel sickness (*see page 130*)
Vomiting and nausea (*see page 117*)

More and more people are travelling abroad for work and holidays, and with that extended travel comes the risk of illnesses that we do not normally come across in the UK. Many conditions are the result of infections contracted by consuming contaminated water or food. Still others are caused by extremes of temperature.

Anyone planning to travel outside Europe, America, Canada, Australia and New Zealand will probably need immunisations before departure. Check with your doctor for individual requirements.

(*See* **First Aid Kit for the Traveller**, *page 164*)

# USEFUL ADDRESSES

In an emergency, you can call the **police**, **ambulance**, **fire brigade**, or **coastguard** on **999** or **112**

**Childline**
0800 1111

**National Drugs Helpline**
0800 776600

**NHS Helpline**
0800 665544
*(for information on health services, operation waiting times, common diseases, emergency numbers)*

**British Allergy Foundation**
Deepdene House
30 Bellegrove Road
Welling
Kent DA16 3BY
0181 303 8583

**British Dental Association**
64 Wimpole Street
London W1H 8AL

**British Diabetic Association**
10 Queen Anne Street
London W1M 0BD
0171 323 1531

**British Heart Foundation**
14 Fitzhardinge Street
London W1H 4DH
0171 935 0185

**Help the Aged**
St James's Walk
Clerkenwell Green
London EC1R 0BE
0171 253 0253

**Miscarriage Association**
Head Office
c/o Clayton Hospital
Northgate
Wakefield
West Yorkshire WF1 3JS
01924 200799

**National Asthma Campaign**
Providence House
Providence Place
London N1 0NT
0171 226 0226

**ROSPA (Royal Society for the Prevention of Accidents)**
Edgbaston Park
353 Bristol Road
Birmingham B5 7ST
0121 248 2000

**St John's Ambulance**
Contact: National Headquarters
St John's Ambulance
Edwina Mountbatten House
63 York Street
London W1H 1PS
0171 258 3456
*(for information on their First Aid courses)*

# INDEX

## EMERGENCIES AND TREATMENTS

# INDEX OF SYMPTOMS

This index is intended as an aid to diagnosis. The list of symptoms is not exhaustive.

# PICTURE CREDITS

t = top   m = middle   b = bottom   r = right   l = left

Paul Lawrence
Pages: 11, 20, 23 t, 31 tl&r, 41 bl&r, 42 br, 45, 50, 51, 55, 59 t, 60, 63, 64, 67, 69, 70 br, 73, 81, 87, 88, 90, 91, 92, 96, 97, 98, 102, 103 tl&r, 108, 109, 110, 111, 112, 115 bl&r, 118, 119, 120, 121, 124, 125, 126, 131, 132, 134, 135, 136, 137, 138, 139, 140, 141 bl&r, 142, 143, 144, 145, 146, 147, 148, 150, 151, 152, 153, 154, 155, 156, 157, 158, 159

William de la Hey
Pages: 10, 14, 21, 22, 24, 25, 26, 29, 30, 32, 33, 36, 37, 40, 41 tr, 44, 47, 48, 54 tl&b, 57, 58, 59 br, 65, 66, 68, 78, 79, 80, 82, 83, 84, 85, 86, 93, 94, 95, 105, 107, 113, 122, 127, 133, 141 tl, 160,163

Victoria Upton
Pages: 23 b, 28, 31 bl&r , 38, 39, 42 tl, 53, 70 tl, 74

The Image Bank
Pages: 54 tr, 75, 115 tr

Jalite UK Ltd
Page: 16

Kidde Thorn Fire Protection Ltd
Page:15

National Medical Slide Bank
Page: 100

Oxford Scientific Films
Page: 116 l&r

The Royal Botanic Gardens, Kew
Page: 103 bl&r

Science Photo Library
Pages: 171 t&b, 172 t&b

Zefa Pictures Ltd
Page: 12, 165